Sentience and Animal Welfare

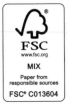

Sentience and Animal Welfare

Donald M. Broom

Professor of Animal Welfare (Emeritus)
Centre for Anthrozoology and Animal Welfare
Department of Veterinary Medicine
and St Catharine's College
University of Cambridge, UK

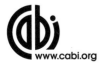

www.cabi.org

CABI is a trading name of CAB International

CABI
Nosworthy Way
Wallingford
Oxfordshire OX10 8DE
UK

Tel: +44 (0)1491 832111
Fax: +44 (0)1491 833508
E-mail: info@cabi.org
Website: www.cabi.org

CABI
38 Chauncy Street
Suite 1002
Boston, MA 02111
USA

Tel: +1 800 552 3083 (toll free)
E-mail: cabi-nao@cabi.org

A catalogue record for this book is available from the British Library, London, UK.

Library of Congress Cataloging-in-Publication Data

Broom, Donald M., author.
  Sentience and animal welfare / Donald M. Broom.
    pages cm.
  Includes bibliographical references and indexes.
  ISBN 978-1-78064-403-5 (hbk : alk. paper) -- ISBN 978-1-78064-404-2 (pbk. : alk. paper) 1. Emotions in animals. 2. Consciousness in animals. 3. Animal welfare. I. Title.
  [DNLM: 1. Animal Welfare. 2. Bioethical Issues. 3. Consciousness. 4. Emotions. 5. Perception. 6. Sensation. HV 4708]

  QL785.27.B76 2014
  591.5--dc23

                     2014006675

ISBN-13: 978 1 78064 403 5 (hbk)
         978 1 78064 404 2 (pbk)

Commissioning editors: Sarah Hulbert and Julia Killick
Editorial assistant: Alexandra Lainsbury
Production editor: Tracy Head

Typeset by SPi, Pondicherry, India.
Printed and bound by CPI Group (UK) Ltd, Croydon, CR0 4YY.

Table of Contents

Preface

People spend much time writing and discussing clever or stupid actions, learning and memory, suffering or feeling happy, and how to deal with the various aspects of the world in which we live. These are the subjects of this book. Sentience is a term used in relation to human questions, such as when a fetus or baby is fully functioning, and how we decide when brain function has been lost in the brain-damaged or old (Chapter 9). However, its most widespread use concerns the abilities of various animal species. How clever are the animals and what can they feel?

An aim of the book is to counter widely stated human prejudices. One is the idea that humans are very different from all other animals. Hence many similarities are described. Another is that mammals have brains that function at a completely different level from those of birds, fish or invertebrate animals such as octopus, squid, lobsters or spiders. The abilities and functioning described in Chapters 4, 5, 6 and 7 on cognition, feelings, awareness and motivation show more close parallels across the range of animals than many people would expect.

A biological interpretation of words is used in the book because serious errors in everyday life can come from misunderstandings when words about body and brain are misused. For example, since people are animals, statements here refer to humans and to non-human animals. The wording: 'humans and other animals' is used rather than 'humans and animals'. The term 'animal' is used erroneously by many people to refer only to mammals, whereas all biologists use 'animal' for birds, fish, insects, molluscs, worms, jellyfish, etc. Also, there is much reference to the brain in this book, but little reference to the mind, because, as explained, there are not two distinct sets of functions and so the word 'mind' is scientifically redundant. There is also explanation of why feelings and knowledge do not come from the heart or the gut. A glossary defining the concepts used in the book is included.

The concept of welfare is of key importance in our lives and in that of other animals. Hence the concept and its history are explained in Chapters 1 and 3, and the rapid developments in animal welfare science are chronicled in Chapter 8. The assessment of welfare and how the methodology is being related to legislation and codes of practice is discussed. As explained in Chapter 11, animal welfare is a part of the sustainability of systems in which we use or have an effect on animals. The increase in the power of consumers in dictating to retail companies, production companies and governments is emphasized. We are moving from a 'push' society driven by producers to a 'pull' society driven by consumers. Members of the European Parliament receive more letters about animal welfare than about any other topic. Other matters discussed in this chapter include the welfare of whales, animal welfare and the World Trade Organization action on seal products, and welfare aspects of the use of genetically modified and cloned animals. Many of the matters considered in this book require ethical decisions. Hence Chapter 2 has discussions of ethics and morality and Chapter 10 is concerned with ethical decisions about human sentience and animal protection.

A wide range of areas of academic research have to be considered in order to adequately discuss the various aspects of sentience, cognition, emotion and animal welfare, with their philosophical, economic and legal components and consequences. As a result, this text cannot be comprehensive in all areas but just presents the various concepts, giving examples of relevant studies. References are therefore made to comprehensive books, as well as to the important papers from which the ideas are derived.

I thank all my colleagues, family and friends who have helped me with this book. In particular I thank Anthony Podberscek, Edmund Rolls, Liz Paul, Marian Dawkins, Melissa Bateson, Mike Mendl, Richard Kirkden and Murray Corke for ideas, and my wife Sally Broom for discussions and help with collecting information. I also thank CABI editorial staff for helping to improve the book.

Donald M. Broom
Centre for Animal Welfare and Anthrozoology
Department of Veterinary Medicine and St Catharine's College
University of Cambridge

Glossary

Abnormal behaviour, Aberrant behaviour: behaviour that differs in pattern, frequency or context from that shown by most members of the species in conditions that allow a full range of behaviour.

Adaptation: (at the individual level) the use of regulatory systems, with their behavioural and physiological components, so as to allow an individual to cope with its environmental conditions.

Affect: feelings, emotions and moods.

Aggression: an act or threat of action, directed by one individual towards another, with the intention of disadvantaging that individual by actually or potentially causing injury, pain or fear.

Allogrooming: grooming directed at another individual animal.

Aversive: such as to cause avoidance or withdrawal.

Awareness: a state during which concepts of environment, of self and of self in relation to environment result from complex brain analysis of sensory stimuli or constructs based on memory.

Causal factor: the inputs to a decision making centre, following interpretation in the light of experience, of a wide variety of external changes and internal states of the body.

Cognition: having a representation in the brain of an object, event or process in relation to others, where the representation can exist whether or not the object, event or process is directly detectable or actually occurring at the time.

Conscious individual: an individual with the capability to perceive and respond to sensory stimuli.

Conspecific: belonging to the same species.

Cope: to cope is to have control of mental and bodily stability.

Depression: a condition of brain and behaviour associated with sagging posture, unresponsiveness and reduced cognitive function.

Dominance: an individual animal is said to be dominant over another when it acts so as to gain priority of access to a resource such as food or a mate. A dominant individual need not be superior in fighting ability to a subordinate.

Emotion: a physiologically describable component of a feeling characterized by electrical and neurochemical activity in particular regions of the brain,

autonomic nervous system activity, hormone release and peripheral consequences including behaviour.

Ethics: the study of moral issues.

Euthanasia: killing an individual for the benefit of that individual and in a
humane way.

Fear: a feeling that occurs when there is perceived to be actual danger or a risk
of danger.

Feedback: the effect of a system output, in response to a system input, which
modifies that input by reducing it (negative feedback) or enhancing it (positive feedback).

Feedforward: the effect of an action which, prior to any input, modifies the
state of the system, usually in such a way that the effect of a subsequent
input is partly or wholly nullified.

Feeling: a brain construct, involving at least perceptual awareness, which is
associated with a life-regulating system, is recognizable by the individual
when it recurs and may change behaviour or act as a reinforcer in learning.

Fitness reduction: this involves increased mortality, or failure to grow or to
reproduce.

A freedom: a possibility for action conferred by one individual or group upon
another.

Functional systems: the different sorts of biological activity in the living
animal that together make up the life process: for example, temperature
regulation, feeding, predator avoidance. These functional systems have
behavioural and physiological components.

Genotype: the genetic constitution of an individual organism designated with
reference either to a single trait or to a set of traits.

Health: the state of an individual as regards its attempts to cope with pathology.

Humane: treatment of animals in such a way that their welfare is good to a
certain high degree.

Humane killing: use of a killing procedure that does not cause poor welfare
and, if there is stunning, a stunning procedure that results in instantaneous
insensibility or, if the agent causing insensibility or death is a gas or injectable substance, no poor welfare occurs before insensibility and then death.

Innovation: this is said to occur when a new solution to a problem, or an
action that meets new requirements, is discovered.

Instinct: a term implying behaviour that is entirely genetically controlled. The
use of this term is undesirable and confusing because neither behaviour nor
any other of the characteristics of a whole animal can develop independently of all environmental influences.

Knowledge: acquired information that can be used subsequently.

Learning: a change in the brain that results in behaviour being modified for
longer than a few seconds, as a consequence of information from outside the
brain.

Metacognition: this means to know what you know.

Mind: not defined, as the term is best avoided in a scientific context.

Mood: a brain state that often involves feelings, continues for more than a few minutes and influences decision making and behaviour.

Moral: pertaining to right rather than to wrong.

Motivation: the process within the brain that controls which behaviours and physiological changes occur and when.

Motivational state: a combination of the levels of all causal factors.

Need: a requirement, which is part of the basic biology of an animal, to obtain a particular resource or to respond to a particular environmental or bodily stimulus.

Obligation: a duty to act, or to refrain from acting, in a way that potentially affects another individual.

Pain: an aversive sensation and feeling associated with actual or potential tissue damage.

Pathology: the detrimental derangement of molecules, cells and functions that occurs in living organisms in response to injurious agents or deprivations

Phenotype: the observable properties of an organism as they have developed under the combined influences of the genetic constitution of the individual and the effects of environmental factors.

Play: carrying out a movement or intellectual process, either in the absence of its usual objective or by using an inefficient means of achieving a goal, solely in order to engage in that movement or process.

Quality of life: welfare during a period of more than a few days.

Reciprocal altruism: this occurs when an altruistic act by individual A, directed towards individual B, is followed by some equivalent act by B directed towards A; or by an act directed towards A whose occurrence is made more likely by the presence or behaviour of B.

Reflex: a simple response involving the central nervous system but not higher brain centres and occurring very shortly after the stimulus that evokes it.

Reinforcer: an environmental change which increases or decreases the likelihood that an animal will make a particular response, i.e. a reward (positive reinforcer) or a punishment (negative reinforcer).

Right: a legal entitlement which can be defended using the laws of the country, or a privilege which is justifiable on moral grounds. The moral grounds may be religious.

Self-awareness: the cognitive process in an individual when it identifies and has a concept of its body or possessions as being its own so that it can discriminate these from non-self stimuli.

Selfish: this describes an individual acting in a way that increases its fitness at the expense of the fitness of one or more other individuals while being aware of the likely effects on itself and on the harmed individual or individuals.

Sentience: having the awareness and cognitive ability necessary to have feelings (for more detail see **Sentient being**).

Sentient being: one that has some ability: (i) to evaluate the actions of others in relation to itself and third parties; (ii) to remember some of its own actions and their consequences; (iii) to assess risks and benefits; (iv) to have some feelings; and (v) to have some degree of awareness.

Stereotypy: a repeated, relatively invariate sequence of movements which has no obvious function.

Stimulation: the effect of one or more stimuli on an individual animal or part of it.

Stimulus: an environmental change which excites one or more receptors or other parts of the nervous system of an animal.

Stress: an environmental effect on an individual which over-taxes its control systems and results in adverse consequences and eventually reduced fitness.

Suffering: one or more bad feelings continuing for more than a few seconds or minutes.

Sustainable: a system or procedure is sustainable if it is acceptable now and if its expected future effects are acceptable, in particular in relation to resource availability, consequences of functioning and morality of action.

Welfare: the state of an individual as regards its attempts to cope with its environment.

The Qualities That Make Up Sentience

1

1.1   Why Are We Interested in Sentience?

People have always wondered what is the essential quality that makes us human. We differ from inanimate objects in that we are alive: breathing by using oxygen and producing carbon dioxide; metabolizing using a variety of enzyme systems; repairing the body; sometimes growing and reproducing. The basic aspects of these capabilities we share with other animals and plants. However, people have always sought a means of differentiating ourselves from other organisms. The plants, at least most of them, have the great advantage of being able to produce energy from sunlight using chlorophyll, so we share an inadequacy with other animals. Most people do not appreciate that we are inadequate in comparison with plants and assume that animals are superior. Starting from this premise, our major perceived rivalry is with other animal species. We share a wide range of capabilities with vertebrate and invertebrate animals, such as digesting, locomotion, sensory functioning and brain control of a variety of processes. Some of the details of these abilities have been known to people for a million years or more. As explained in later chapters, observations of behaviour indicate that, while we have knowledge of the functioning of other animals, many other animals also appreciate that individuals of their own and other species need air, food and other resources.

In order to promote the idea that people are special in some way, efforts have been made to describe unique qualities. It was difficult to do this because of our great similarity to other species. Hence somewhat nebulous concepts of the essence of humanity were devised. In human societies, a soul or a psyche or a spirit is attributed to people, or at least to some people. It is often emphasized that humans have 'free will' and it is assumed that other animals do not, or at least have much less of it. The view is based on prejudice, as it is obvious from observations of behaviour that most animals are far from being automata with no control of their lives. While soul, psyche, spirit and free will are qualities of individuals, they might also be shared to some degree with others, or linked to a concept of God. When Descartes wrote about individuals having a social spirit he was making a biological and a religious statement. This idea is discussed further in Chapter 2 and has been developed, by the author and others, in books about the biological basis for morality and religion (Ridley, 1996; de Waal, 1996; Broom, 2003).

The soul, psyche or spirit of a person has many components that are also thought of as components of sentience. Although the idea of sentience is more recent, it fulfils some of the same functions as the older ideas, especially when used to refer to humans rather than non-humans. When Descartes referred to the spirit, which he and others have sometimes called soul or mind, he considered it to be separate from the body (see for example Rowlands, 2012, 2013). While the spirit implied connection to others, the soul or mind was the individual part of the spirit. What is the mind? Biologists would now say that behaviour, and some of the physiological functioning of the body, is controlled by the brain. An individual's perception, cognition, awareness and feelings occur in the brain of that individual and are the consequence of, or cause of, the functioning of sensory mechanisms, muscular responses, glandular responses and other bodily changes. The organs of the body – for example the heart – will influence brain function, but thoughts and feelings are in the brain and not in the heart or any other part of the body. With this role of the brain established, it is not useful for the concept of mind to be considered separately from the brain (Broom, 2003), except perhaps where it means the same as soul, or a component of spirit, and refers to links among individuals.

Dictionary definitions of sentient refer to: (i) feeling or being capable of feeling; or (ii) being able to exercise the senses and respond to sensory stimuli (Merriam Webster, 2005; *Concise Oxford English Dictionary*, 2011). Most early usage of the term sentience (see Section 1.3) implied that the individual has the level of awareness and associated brain function that makes it possible to have positive and negative feelings. DeGrazia (1996) refers to a sentient being as one that is capable of having feelings. He develops this idea, quoting Sapontzis (1987) who argues that there is no point in an individual having the capacity for feeling unless they can recognize, desire and pursue pleasure and avoid pain. DeGrazia also considers that sentience does not 'make sense' without conation, that is, having a drive to perform acts, with or without knowledge of the origin of that drive; and conation does not 'make sense' without sentience. Kirkwood (2006) also considers that sentience is the capacity to feel something. Webster (2010) does not define sentience but he says that 'a sentient animal has feelings that matter'. He explains what matters to animals in terms of strength of preference studies.

When the words sentient, aware, conscious, emotion and feeling are used, they are often used together. Efforts to define or explain one of these terms often involve the use of the others. This is because it is difficult to find other descriptive, definitive words. For example Le Doux (1995), writing about emotion, says 'a subjective emotional experience, like the feeling of being afraid, results when we become consciously aware of an emotion system of the brain like the defense system'. As in most of the writing about these subjects, his focus is on humans. It is assumed that the reader will understand what is meant when 'subjective' is used, will appreciate what a feeling is and will recall being consciously aware and afraid. When other people are discussed, our empathy for them and some observations that we can make lead us to believe that their brain processes are very similar to ours. If another animal species is considered, we have some empathy, but may have doubts about it. Also, we may have a more limited set of observations of the behaviour of that species, and may have been told either that animals of that kind have very different brain structure, or that they are very similar to us. Hence we may or may not conclude that processes like those of humans occur in the brain of such an animal. The prejudices of those in the academic community may well be the reason why many scientists are not willing to say that non-human animals can be conscious, aware or have feelings.

A major change in attitudes to the idea of awareness and feelings in non-human animals has occurred as studies of behaviour have become more detailed. In addition, brain mechanisms have been studied using new methods such as brain recording and scanning: electroencephalography (EEG), positron-emission tomography (PET-scanning), magneto-encephalography (MEG) and frequency-modulated magnetic resonance imaging (fMRI). For some methods now, and for other methods during most of the time since their development, these scanning procedures required that the individual be immobile inside or attached to laboratory apparatus. This precluded their use for freely moving animals and was too frightening to the animals to allow useful studies. Only largely automatic mechanisms could be investigated. This situation is just starting to change as new methods are developed.

One anomaly in the writings of biological scientists (pointed out by Rollin, 1989) has been that while many were unwilling to attribute feelings such as pain and anxiety to any species other than man, laboratory animals have been used for many years as models for humans in work on pain and anxiety. Most scientists would say that a substantial part of the mechanisms involved in pain and anxiety exist in mice and other laboratory species, but that there is some key difference in higher processing. However, this key difference is assumed not to invalidate the application of the laboratory results to humans.

It is assumed that people are sentient, but when did humans or their fore-bears become sentient? The idea that some races of people alive now differ significantly from others in their level of brain function is now known to be incorrect. Also, there is no evidence for differences between races in sensory abilities and feelings, for example capacity to feel pain. The range of human ability within each race is much greater than the range across races. Similarly, the idea that early humans were primitive in every way and very different from modern humans is not supported by written or archaeological evidence. Bronze Age people in Eastern Britain 4000 years ago (e.g. Flag Fen near Peterborough) were living in complex communities, using boats and trading goods with people on the other side of the English Channel. Paintings by people who lived a million years ago indicate sophisticated social living and a good understanding of the environment. Sentience would seem to have existed in people throughout the ages. The question of when sentience arises during development, and when it is lost due to pathology, injury or senility is considered in Chapter 9.

1.2   How Do People View Species Perceived to be Like Us or Unlike Us?

When people have the concept that they have a soul, or have sentience, there will be discussion about whether or not other groups of people, or other kinds of animals, have that quality. There is a widespread tendency to identify more with some species than with others because of their obvious, human-like characteristics. If the body form and behaviour of an animal are similar to those of humans, that animal is more likely to be respected and more likely to be judged to have a soul or to be sentient. Qualities often perceived to indicate that the animal species deserves respect include possession of a relatively flat face, hands, a distinct head, vocalizations ranging in pitch, fur or hair, body length of 1–2 m, warm blood, red blood, lack of body armour and relative uniformity of tooth size. These judgements are related to biological qualities of the animal species but do not always take account of biology in the way that a scientist would evaluate it. It is obvious that similarity to human form and function is an important aspect of this judgement. However, similarity to animals used by man as companions is another aspect. Being a species regarded as dangerous to man or being thought of as a pest make an animal less likely to be respected.

The more different from humans an animal appears to be, the less likely it is to be evaluated as sentient. This is one reason why fish, reptiles such as snakes, insects, spiders and molluscs tend to receive little human respect. However, another category of animals that are respected less than might be expected from their anatomy and behaviour, are those that people keep so they can eat them. In order to be able to eat animals, many people feel that they must denigrate and devalue them by saying that they are stupid or are in some way less similar to humans than they really are. Farm animals have long been misrepresented in this way in human writing and media.

These attitudes to animals are translated into law and codes of practice so animals perceived to be human-like are protected more than those that are not (see Chapter 10). However, there has been a change in laws in recent years, because biological information is becoming more important in decisions about laws and unscientific prejudice is becoming less important. The European Union (EU) Treaty of Lisbon (European Union, 2007) says in the course of a statement about animal protection and welfare (Article 6b), 'since animals are sentient beings...'. This wording had the intention to protect the animals commonly used by man, for example on farms, in the laboratory, or as companions, but actually refers to all animals. The term animal refers to flatworms, flies and snails as much as it refers to parrots, dogs and chimpanzees. A question that is raised (Kirkwood, 2006) is whether or not we should give equal protection to a dog and to the fleas on a dog. Part of the aim of this book is to explain the evidence about the components of sentience in a wide range of animals and in humans, ranging from a fertilized egg to a functioning adult, or to a scarcely functioning brain-damaged adult.

1.3   The Concept of Sentience

Animals vary in the extent to which they are aware of themselves (DeGrazia, 1996) and of their interactions with their environment, including their ability to experience pleasurable states such as happiness and aversive states such as pain, fear and grief. This capacity may be referred to as their degree of sentience. As explained above, the term 'sentience' has generally been used to mean that the individual has the capacity to have feelings: that is, sentience means having the awareness and cognitive ability necessary to have feelings. This raises the question of what abilities are needed in order to have this capacity. Sentience implies a range of abilities, not just having feelings. A definition, slightly modified from Broom (2006c), is: a sentient being is one that has some ability: (i) to evaluate the actions of others in relation to itself and third parties; (ii) to remember some of its own actions and their consequences; (iii) to assess risks and benefits; (iv) to have some feelings; and (v) to have some degree of awareness. The various aspects of this definition will be explained in this chapter and addressed in the remainder of this book.

The definition of sentient being stated above enlarges on the short definition of sentience as 'having the capacity to feel' by Kirkwood (2006). However, Kirkwood also says 'to be sentient is to have a feeling of something'. I do not agree that an individual is only sentient when having a feeling, and also think that to be sentient is more than just having feelings. Neither do I find it helpful to say, as Kirkwood does, that sentience is something that we experience; or, as in some definitions, to include having simple perceptions as an alternative meaning of sentience.

Human opinion as to which individuals of our own and other species are sentient has generally changed over time in well-educated societies to encompass first all humans, instead of just a subset of humans, and then certain mammals that were kept as companions; animals which seemed most similar to humans such as monkeys; the larger mammals; all mammals; all warm-blooded animals; then all vertebrates; and now some invertebrates.

People have long appreciated the sentience of various domestic and other well-known animals and have often thought of their dog or horse as an example to follow or a friend who would help, rather than just as a resource object. However, a rabbit is viewed differently according to whether it is a family pet, a laboratory animal, an animal kept for meat production, or a wild animal that eats your crops. This is not scientifically sound. A rabbit is a rabbit and each one feels pain or has cognitive function (Broom, 2007a).

1.4   Definitions and Descriptions of Components of Sentience

Key issues in any discussion of the sentience of all animals, including fish and invertebrates, are: (i) whether they are aware of what is happening around them; (ii) whether they are capable of cognitive processing; and (iii) whether they can have feelings such as pain. The meaning of awareness is discussed in Chapter 6. A definition by Broom (1998) is modified here: awareness is a state during which concepts of environment, of self, and of self in relation to environment result from complex brain analysis of sensory stimuli or constructs based on memory. Its existence can be deduced using careful observation, generally in controlled, experimentally contrived situations. The information obtained can help us to understand which of the several levels of awareness is indicated (Sommerville and Broom, 1998). A conscious individual is one that has the capability to perceive and respond to sensory stimuli. This is essentially the definition of Blood and Studdert (1988): 'capable of responding to sensory stimuli; awake; aware'.

As explained further in Chapter 9, animals are more likely to be considered sentient if they can learn much, learn fast and make few errors once they have learned. These abilities are the basis of evaluating the actions of other individuals and remembering actions and their consequences. For any individual, assessing risk and benefit is also an important part of appreciating its environment in a way that allows some control of interactions with it. Learning is a change in the brain, which results in behaviour being modified for longer than a few seconds, as a consequence of information from outside the brain (Broom and Johnson, 1993). These topics are discussed in detail in Chapters 4, 5 and 6. As discussed further in Chapter 4, cognition is having a representation in the brain of an object, event or process in relation to others, where the representation can exist whether or not the object, event or process is directly detectable or actually occurring at the time.

The ability to feel pain and some forms of pleasure are generally included among the capabilities of sentient animals. A feeling is a brain construct, involving at least perceptual awareness, which is associated with a life-regulating system, is recognizable by the individual when it recurs and may change behaviour or act as a reinforcer in learning (Broom, 1998). The concept of 'emotion' overlaps with that of 'feeling'. As discussed at length in Chapter 5, emotion is describable using physiological measures.

As explained by Broom (2003), the reluctance of scientists to attribute complex abilities and feelings to non-humans has slowed the development of our knowledge of sophisticated brain function in non-humans. Researchers have been unwilling to carry out studies in the area because, if they used words such as awareness, feeling, emotion and mood, they risked the scorn of other scientists and having difficulties in future in obtaining research funding and getting papers published.

Ethics, Morality and Attitudes   2

2.1   Ethics

Something is moral if it pertains to right rather than to wrong. The question of what is right, or good, or beneficial is discussed further by Broom (2003). However, as Midgley (1994) has emphasized, morality should not be thought of as a topic that is obscure and difficult to comprehend. We each have many clear ideas about actions that are good or not good. Most people would agree that behaving morally involves judging right and wrong and behaving accordingly (Planalp, 1999). Hence decisions about moral issues are taken many times during every day. People 'behave morally' most of the time and often discuss questions of what is right or wrong. In doing this they express an interest in ethics which is the study of moral issues. Determining what is moral is sometimes very obvious but, at other times, involves considerable thought. While several capabilities have arisen during evolution that promote moral behaviour, the idea that ethics can be entirely based on 'uneducated gut feelings' is not supported by most people, and is clearly not a logical and reliable guide to conduct.

Whether or not something has moral value is an ethical question. Do individual people, non-human animals, plants and inanimate objects have value? If they do, what kind of value do they have? A value that derives from usefulness is sometimes called instrumental value. The objects in a person's house have value in relation to how much that person wants to use them, and a dog has value according to how much it is used as a companion, as a stimulus to exercise, etc. However, most people also think of value in relation to convertibility to a general resource such as money, and this may or may not correspond with how much an object or animal is used. One meaning of value, different from value as a resource, is value in an absolute or intrinsic sense. When most of us think of a person or of a dog known to us, we consider that the person or dog has a value independent of utility to ourselves. The kind of value ascribed to an animal will be different according to how concepts such as 'we have dominion over animals' are used (see Broom, 2003). If dominion is taken to mean that the animals exist only for human benefit, their value will vary according to human use, and their welfare will be important only if it affects use. If dominion means stewardship and obligation to care for each individual, the animals have intrinsic value, and those who use them have an obligation to avoid poor welfare in those animals. As Hiebert (1996) has pointed out, those who wrote in the Old Testament of the Bible about dominion over nature, including animals, had much less possibility for control than people today have. The stewardship approach to animals is much more in line with modern ethics.

A further relevant relationship is that between individuals having value and individuals as property. Can one person be the property of another? The widely held view nowadays is that they cannot. Can an animal be the property of a person? In one sense, most would say 'yes', but does property mean the same for a cow and a coat? Both might be bought and sold, but while the coat could be cut in pieces, a live cow could not. The person has no obligation to the coat but does have the obligation to provide for the needs of the cow. For some people, the obligations to the cow cease when the cow is dead. For other people those obligations continue after death in that they consider it wrong to eat the cow and wrong to keep a cow solely in order to eat it.

One issue, considered in this and later chapters, is the extent to which sentience or lack of it might alter value. A second issue is how the value placed on an individual might alter our treatment of and concern about the welfare of the individual.

2.2 Morality, Selfishness and Altruism

Morality is part of most aspects of our lives. Every person has ideas about what is right and some actions are considered to be right by a very high proportion of people. People take account of morality in their actions and moral issues are a frequent topic of discussion. However, some people do not think of morality as an issue with a biological basis. If it does have a biological basis, as several authors have argued (Kropotkin, 1902; Kummer, 1978; de Waal, 1996; Ridley, 1996; Broom, 2003, 2006c), there will be links between the functioning of humans and non-humans in relation to decisions about which actions to carry out because they are moral and which to avoid because they are not.

There are many ideas that biologists would take as axiomatic, for example that humans are animals, but which some other people would not readily accept. Another example is that the organ involved in decision making in humans and other animals is their brain and that the heart is not directly involved in decision making. These and many other biological facts are relevant to the discussions about the biological basis of morality that are presented here.

Some people would not accept the topic of morality as suitable for discussion from a biological perspective, because it is thought of as sacred or God-given. It has been argued that the facts of nature should not be related to human values (Moore, 1903). Even some biologists regard morality as in some way outside biology (Dawkins, 1976; Alexander, 1979; Williams, 1988).

The idea of the 'selfish gene', proposed by Richard Dawkins (1976) in a book that was valuable in promoting the understanding of genetic and behavioural mechanisms, is misleading. 'Selfish describes an individual acting in a way that increases its fitness at the expense of the fitness of one or more other individuals whilst being aware of the likely effects on itself and on the harmed individual or individuals' (Broom, 2003). The word selfish is thus limited to individuals with awareness so it could not describe a gene. If a word is widely used with one set of connotations, it cannot be transferred to another set without causing the reader or hearer to misunderstand either the breadth of its implications or the concept itself (Midgley, 1994). A problem that results from Dawkins' usage of 'selfish gene' is that people may argue that we are not responsible for the effects of our genes, that genes are often selfish, and hence that there is nothing wrong with being selfish. A better term to use in referring to genes that promote the fitness of the bearer (i.e. the actions benefit the subject at the expense of others that are harmed by the action) is 'harmful subject-benefit' (Broom, 2003).

In order to explain the basis for morality we often refer to altruism. An altruistic act by an individual is one that involves some cost to that individual in terms of reduced fitness but increases the fitness of one or more other individuals. Reciprocal altruism is defined here as occurring when an altruistic act by individual A, directed towards individual B, is followed by some equivalent act by B directed towards A or by an act directed towards A whose occurrence is made more likely by the presence or behaviour of B.

Animals that live in social groups, including humans in groups, cooperate in many ways that benefit the cooperating individuals more than would occur if they just competed with one another. Those who have watched stable groups of cattle, horses or various primate species will have observed allogrooming. The individual groomed will often, at a later time, groom the groomer. In all species, some body areas are difficult for the individual itself to groom efficiently and, where mutual grooming occurs, ectoparasite infestation tends to be less. Benham, reported by Broom and Fraser (2007), describes mutual grooming relationships in unrelated cows in suckler herds. These cows spend much time together and seldom show aggression to one another.

There are many ways in which individuals can gain more food by responding to or collaborating with others. Broom (1981a) lists:

• joining others who are likely to have found food;
• observing others in order to find food sources or to learn how to acquire food;

- collaborating in hunting for food;
- collaborating in acquiring food;
- collaborating in handling and defending food;
- collaborating in avoiding depleted food sources;
- sharing food; and
- giving food to others.

Wolves, pelicans and crocodiles are among the species described as collaborating in obtaining food. Vampire bats, ravens and chimpanzees are among those that share food (de Waal, 1989; Broom, 2003).

In addition to the more obvious kinds of cooperation, the commonest kind of altruistic behaviour in social groups, which is often reciprocated, is to avoid injuring other individuals (Broom, 2003). Great care is usually, although not always, taken by individuals in social groups:

- to avoid collisions, thus benefitting the avoider as well as the avoided;
- not to step on others;
- not to injure them with horns or teeth;
- not to push others out of trees, or over cliffs; and
- not to put others in danger from predators.

Cattle, for example those in Fig. 2.1, could easily injure one another but move around in such a way that they do not. If any accidental harm to another does occur, this can be followed by changed behaviour on the part of the harmed individual, others in the social group and the one who has harmed. Harm may be followed by some form of retribution, but either accidental or deliberate harm may also be followed by reconciliation, at least in primates (de Waal, 1996). The individuals which take part in reconciliation may form alliances in order to achieve social and other objectives. Bonobos have been found to share food with strangers when a social interaction could occur and also to help strangers to obtain food (Tan and Hare, 2013).

Once altruism occurs and is reciprocated, the possibility of cheating becomes important. A variety of characteristics of individuals, any of which would tend to promote altruistic and moral behaviour, is listed in Table 2.1. Among these are ways of detecting and responding to individuals who cheat, in that they fail to avoid harming others, or make no effort to reciprocate to an individual, or to contribute in a more general way within a group if benefit is received.

The characteristics listed in Table 2.1 are discussed further in Section 2.4. Feelings are important parts of the mechanisms that individuals use in order to cope with the various problems of life. The ways in which natural selection might have acted to promote moral actions is discussed by Broom (2006c) and the role of religion in supporting moral actions by Broom (2003).

As explained by Broom (2011), social animals such as humans have evolved characteristics that make them responsive to others in their societies

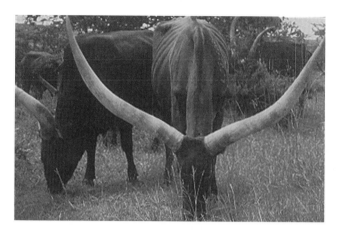

Fig. 2.1. Cattle like this, with horns that could easily harm others in their social group, go through almost all of their lives taking care not to harm others (photograph D.M. Broom).

Table 2.1. Individual characteristics that may promote altruistic or moral behaviour (modified after Broom, 2003).

1	Affection for certain types of individuals, where this affection reduces the chances that harm will be done to them. The individuals may be close relatives, or group members, or those perceived to be likely to be in one of those categories
2	Affection for the same individuals as in 1 above, where that affection increases the likelihood of carrying out behaviour that is beneficial to them
3	Ability to recognize individuals that might be beneficiaries or benefactors
4	Ability to remember the actions of others that resulted in benefit to oneself or to others in the group
5	Ability to remember one's own actions that resulted in a benefit to another individual
6	Ability to assess risk or benefit of own and other actions and either to compare these or to avoid high risk and try to attain high benefit
7	Ability to detect and evaluate cheating
8	Ability to punish or facilitate the punishment of those who cheat
9	Ability to support a social structure that encourages cooperation and discourages cheating
10	Having a desire to conform

in a way that promotes dutiful preferences and actions. This deontological position has arisen in every human society and the mechanisms involved have parallels in other animal societies. Other evolved characteristics increase abilities to assess consequences of actions and to evaluate costs and benefits, i.e. some utilitarian decisions.

People will often avoid actions that could harm others, even if only they know about the action (Gert, 1988; Broom, 2006a). However, they are more likely to refrain from causing harm if those in their social group may come to know about what they have done. As human societies have expanded their contacts, the group that is in moral contact with an individual expanded from the family to the tribe, and has subsequently expanded further to include much larger communities. The communication explosion in the 20th and 21st centuries has resulted in information about the actions of particular people becoming known across the world. As a consequence, it has become harder for harmful actions to be concealed (Broom, 2003). The spread of information about particular actions, and of all knowledge, has been greatly facilitated and has led to an increase in moral behaviour by individuals and, more belatedly, by commercial organizations and nations.

The level of sophistication of the functioning of individuals has often been a factor in decisions about whether or not they are a subject of moral actions. The ways in which human and other animal brains work were a mystery to all people until information became available from relatively recent developments in neurobiology. Our language has not kept pace with these changes, so people make statements about having feelings or knowing something in their heart or in their gut, when all are in the brain. The study of behaviour and of how the brain controls it, and of the great similarities in the physiology of all people and a wide range of other species, has been revolutionary in its impact on human attitudes (Dennett, 1984). Until recently it was really believed by many people: (i) that women had very inferior functioning as compared with men; (ii) that the cognitive ability of people with brown or black skin was less than that of white people; and (iii) that there was an enormous gap in ability and functioning between humans and other species. A wide range of studies now show these views to be wrong. The group of individuals that is respected, in that harm would not normally be caused to its members, has been extended to include humans of all nations and races and to many other animal species. To some extent this is a consequence of information that is available from the media. The person watching a television programme and seeing a parrot, or squirrel, or dog, or pig, or sheep, or raven solve complex problems, may not in future think of that kind of animal as an object, or as a being of no consequence. That person may well become much less likely to directly harm the animal, or to condone harm by others.

2.3 Obligations

Most people have the view that each of us has obligations to others. An obligation is a duty to act, or to refrain from acting, in a way that potentially affects another individual. In my view, this is the best approach to all moral issues and is better than claiming rights or freedoms. Obligations to others might exist because the subject is considered to have an intrinsic value, or because of concern for its welfare (Broom, 2003, 2006b, 2010a).

Moral actions are directed more towards those identified as 'us' than towards those considered to be 'them' (Broom, 2003, 2006a). Categories included as 'us' may be: (i) individuals readily recognized as close relatives; (ii) all of those who know who I am; (iii) those who might have access to some of the same information that I have; or (iv) sentient beings who share characteristics with me. Increased communication efficiency is revolutionizing our degree of concern for other humans and extending our area of moral concern to other species. Companion animals will be in category (i) for some people. Serpell and Paul (1994) found many pet owners stated that they regarded their pets as part of their family. Most pet owners would include their pet in category (ii). All people who consider animals to be sentient, or who know that most mammals have over 90% of the same genes as humans, would include some or many non-human animals in categories (iii) or (iv). In many societies, education levels are now high and there is easy access to good-quality information about people in other countries and about animals whose abilities are complex. Hence there will be a continuing decline in the likelihood that people will cause, or tolerate, poor welfare in foreign people or in animals perceived to be sentient. It is of particular interest that the changes in attitudes to humans and to non-human animals appear to be linked more closely to the education level of people than to their affluence. In countries where the people are relatively poor, but well educated, interest in human and animal welfare has changed in much the same way as in rich countries where people are well educated. The people are willing to incur some degree of financial loss rather than benefit from poor welfare in animals.

If we use a living animal in a way that gives us some benefit, we have some obligations to that animal. One obligation is to avoid causing poor welfare in the animal, except where the action leads to a net benefit to that animal, or to other animals including humans, or to the environment. A utilitarian approach is not sufficient to determine all obligations, however, and a deontological approach is also needed because there are some degrees of poor welfare that are never justified by benefit to others.

Many living organisms are used by humans and many others are affected by human activities. Every living organism is likely to be the subject of more reverence than an inanimate object because living organisms are qualitatively different from inanimate objects in complexity, potential and aesthetic quality. This can affect decisions about whether to kill the organism and whether to conserve such an organism. As a consequence of their ability to respond and behave, we consider that we have more obligations to animals than to microorganisms or plants. We feel concerned about their welfare, especially in the case of the more complex animals (Broom, 2003). Which kinds of animal deserve such consideration (Broom, 2007a, 2010a)? New knowledge has tended to show that the abilities and functioning of non-human animals are more complex than had previously been assumed, so it is my opinion that some reappraisal of the threshold levels for protection is needed. Proposals for change in which animals should be protected have been made by the European Food Safety Authority (EFSA) (2005).

The first question for some of the people who are deciding about the animals that should be protected because their welfare is an important consideration is whether or not the animals are useful. Other arguments about which animals to protect have involved analogy with humans, in that if the animals seem to be more like us they are considered to be more worthy of protection. The argument advocated here (Broom, 2006b) views the qualities of the animal on an absolute scale that includes known animals, but would also be relevant to unknown living beings such as those that might be found on another planet. Such arguments can be supported by scientific evidence (Table 2.2) and this has increased more and more in recent years. This evidence is considered in the remainder of this book.

The most widely accepted obligation to the animals that we use concerns avoidance of poor welfare. As a consequence, learning about animal welfare and its scientific basis is very important for all who have frequent contact with animals.

2.4 Rights

It is my view (Broom, 2003) that all human behaviour and laws should be based on the obligations of each person to act in an acceptable way towards each other person and to each animal that is used. It is better for strategies for living to be based on our obligations rather than to involve the concept of rights. This is because many so-called rights can result in harm to others. A right is a legal entitlement, which can be defended using the laws of the country, or a privilege that is justifiable on moral, perhaps religious, grounds. There are occasions when people state that they have a right to say what they want, or drive as fast as they want, or carry a gun, or select the sex or genetic make-up of their children (Broom, 2006b). In each of these cases the action could cause harms to others. These harms would be accepted by very few people. The argument based on a concept

Table 2.2. Evidence that can be used to decide which animals should be protected (after Broom, 2007a).

1	Complexity of life and behaviour
2	Learning ability
3	Functioning of the brain and nervous system
4	Indications of pain or distress
5	Studies illustrating the biological basis of suffering and other feelings such as fear and anxiety
6	Indications of awareness based on observations and experimental work

of rights can lead to a morally wrong or questionable outcome. Arguments based on the obligation of one individual towards others do not suffer from such problems. This is the reason for my conclusion that the concept of rights is not the best to use and that each person should always focus on how they ought to behave. As far as animal rights are concerned, non-human animals do not normally have legal rights. On the other hand, there are many statements, codes of conduct, or widely accepted but unwritten rules that explain the obligations towards animals of people who use those animals.

2.5   Freedom

The argument presented above criticizing the use of the term 'rights' is also applicable to references to the freedom that an individual asserts, or that is supposed to be given to an individual. Spinoza said that to be free is to act in accordance with necessity. If an individual is subject to a constraint, usually imposed by other persons, and this constraint prevents such action, the individual is not free. A freedom is a possibility for action conferred by one individual or group upon another (Broom, 2003).

People who are kept captive, or who are prevented from obtaining what they need because of other imposed constraints, have significant problems. The restriction or deprivation has negative effects. An extreme example of this is slavery where enslaved individuals have little control over what happens to themselves; another individual, the owner of the slave, has that control. To a somewhat lesser degree, a despotic ruler, or feudal lord, or factory owner, or work-camp supervisor could prevent the needs of the people whom they control from being fulfilled and this would result in poor welfare in those people. The action of placing such constraints on others is wrong and the imposers of the constraints are not fulfilling their obligations to the people for whom they are responsible.

There are people who are imprisoned because of criminal acts, or because there is a high probability that they will endanger others or themselves. There is also restriction of children during their development with the aim of protecting them and helping them to adapt to the society in which they will live. Hence some constraint by some persons on other persons is accepted. This acceptance is on the grounds that the individuals constrained are not fully able to take the decisions that are needed about how to fulfil their own needs yet remain in society. The argument in relation to people in general, to children and to vulnerable people is that they should not be unreasonably subject to constraint or deprivation. However, this argument is sometimes turned around in constitutional documents and in public statements to say that there should be freedom for each individual to do what they want. This is a dangerous argument that should never be accepted without qualification. To argue for freedom in the sense of release from tyranny is civilized. To argue for freedom in the general sense is a recipe for personal and societal disaster.

As stated above in relation to people asserting rights, there are also those who assert that they should have freedom to do what they want. The individual could be asserting that he should be free to do something that is harmful to others; for example to be free to take possessions, or defraud, or injure, or risk causing injury by carrying a gun, or pass on a disease, or decide not to have a child that would be female. Each individual has obligations to others and these obligations inevitably and at all times limit freedom of action. Unqualified assertions that individuals should have freedom of action are illogical and morally wrong.

The arguments presented in relation to humans are also relevant to the animals that we use or with which we interact. All species of animals are capable of living in an appropriate environment without human help. They have a repertoire of abilities and an associated set of needs that can be discovered by biological investigation. The animals can look after themselves so they are not like children or mentally impaired humans. However, if we keep them in our conditions for our benefit, we have an obligation to find out their needs, keep them in such a way that those needs are fulfilled and hence to ensure that their welfare is good. As discussed in Chapter 7, knowledge of the great diversity of needs that animals of a particular species have is key to humane treatment of such animals.

Efforts to list the freedoms that should be allowed to the animals that we keep have been of use as a general guide to management, but with the development of information about the needs of animals, it is now possible to be more precise. The 'five freedoms' (Brambell, 1965) are problematical if the wording is considered exactly. For example, 'freedom from pain, injury and disease' for domestic animals is a desirable state and those responsible for animals should aim at it but it is not achievable. Any animal might slip and fall or collide with something and be caused pain and injury. Pathogens may result in disease that could not have been prevented. Similarly, 'freedom from fear and distress' could not be achieved in individuals that have to encounter humans and 'freedom from hunger and thirst' would not be possible unless food and water were available at all times. 'Freedom to express normal behaviour' would include giving the animals the possibility of showing aggression to others and other antisocial behaviours that would be classified as normal. Just as for humans, freedom for the animals should have social limitations. A consequence of these logical inconsistencies is that some of those who use animals may say that they follow the five freedoms approach, knowing that they are not fully achievable and, as a consequence, failing to follow the general guidelines that the five freedoms list. The four welfare principles and 12 criteria proposed, as a development of the five freedoms concept, by the Welfare Quality project (Blokhuis *et al.*, 2010) are a more useful general guideline. However, they also have points such as: 'no disease', 'no injuries' and 'expressing social behaviour' as part of them. They are aimed at particular, housed land animals so some wording is difficult to apply to extensively kept or aquatic animals, for example 'good housing' and 'comfort around resting'. General guides like these should be used only to help in general planning and not for a particular species. For any animal, the best approach to a scheme for ensuring good welfare is to start with details of the needs of animals of that species, as determined from knowledge of their biological functioning and scientific studies of their preferences. Laws and guidelines for animal care, whose aim is to ensure good welfare, should refer to needs rather than to freedoms.

2.6   Brief History of Attitudes to Animals

The idea that animals used by people should not be treated like inanimate possessions, but should be protected from actions that might cause suffering, is very old and widespread in human society. Irrespective of any law, many people have condemned those perceived as being cruel to animals. On the other hand, cruelty was part of some forms of human entertainment. In Europe, laws intended to prevent cruelty to dogs and horses were passed as long as 200 years ago and were gradually extended to other kinds of animals. Most early laws referred to companion animals and working animals but not to farm animals. Some laws protected animals against the forms of animal experimentation that were considered likely to cause substantial pain to the animals. Laws were also passed which proscribed some forms of entertainment involving animals as being cruel but others were still permitted. Laws aimed at preventing poor welfare in animals have become more wide-ranging, both in terms of species and the different animal uses, and have been passed in more and more countries.

Two components of the thinking of those who want to protect animals are empathy and compassion (Würbel, 2009). As Bentham said, people identify with and care about individuals that can suffer, and this is still a widespread view (Dawkins, 1993). The term 'pathocentrism' is used by German-speaking scientists and refers to those who focus especially on suffering. People are more likely to show empathy with those perceived to have a capacity for feelings similar to those of humans. Griffin (1984) referred to 'a deep-seated sympathy for animals as sentient creatures'. People are also likely to show compassion only to those whom they perceive to need compassion.

The treatment of animals is an area in which codes of conduct and descriptions of good practice exist. Even among groups of people whose objective was to kill animals, there have long existed unwritten codes of conduct concerning what actions were, or were not, permissible. For example, as discussed by Serpell (1986, 1989), people using guns and dogs to hunt mammals or birds would expend energy and resources trying to ensure: (i) that animals were shot in a way so they were likely to die quickly; and (ii) that shot animals were found and killed rather than being left to die slowly. These hunters' codes have the objective of avoiding the worst welfare. The same aim has led to efforts to kill animals humanely in slaughterhouses. Codes of practice relating to animals kept for food production and other purposes have been produced by various organizations. In the EU, and in many countries around the world, the first legislation whose aim was to minimize poor welfare concerned the stunning of animals before slaughter. There is an aesthetic component to the motivation behind such legislation, because most people regard the sight of an animal in pain as repugnant. There is also preference for killing methods that do not involve the sight of blood, and animal welfare scientists sometimes have difficulty in arguing for a method of killing that is demonstrably better for the welfare of the animals but is not aesthetically pleasing. For example, the method of killing unwanted day-old domestic chicks that is best for their welfare is to put them into the rapidly revolving blades of a macerator. The handling is minimal and the death is instantaneous. However, members of the public will sometimes not wish to see this method used. The view of aesthetic matters by some members of the public may lead to actions that have negative effects on animals. A further example is the desire of some people to breed brightly coloured or luminous animals. It is my view that the moral position, relating to welfare, should be considered more important than the aesthetic position.

The way in which animals are treated is much affected by the way in which the human user or carer thinks about those animals. The animal may be thought of as an object to be used that is little different from something inanimate. Actions which cause poor welfare in the animals are much more likely, when there is this attitude, than if the animals are considered to be similar in many ways to humans. Hence knowledge of animal functioning tends to engender respect where the animal is sentient, that is to say that the animal has significant capacity for awareness of itself and its relationships with its environment. In recent years, knowledge of animal functioning, particularly of behaviour and physiology, has increased rapidly and has been the subject of much media attention. This is a major reason for increased concern about the welfare of animals.

Public concern about animal welfare has increased in many countries during the last 30 years and especially in the last 10 years. Evidence for this is summarized in Table 2.3.

Members of the public exert influence by letters to government, to other public bodies and commercial organizations, and by statements that appear in

Table 2.3. Evidence for increased concern about animal welfare (from Broom, 1999b).

1	Letters from the public, media coverage
2	References in parliamentary discussions and government statements
3	Requests for scientific evidence concerning animal welfare
4	Activity of scientific and other advisory committees
5	Funding of scientific research on animal welfare
6	Increased teaching and conferences
7	More legislation

the media. Members of the European Parliament report that they receive more letters about animal welfare than about any other topic. Politicians respond by raising the issues, including them in manifestos, seeking scientific information, encouraging further research and teaching, and passing laws.

People who own or work on farms, or other commercial organizations using animals, are influenced by a variety of factors when they are deciding on animal housing and management policies and when they are executing these policies. They will be endeavouring to make a profit so the monetary costs that they incur, and the potential financial returns that they are likely to get for their product, will be factors of major importance to them. A cost to those involved in the animal industry, which may not be fully appreciated by many of them, results from consumers who do not like some aspect of production and refuse to buy the product (Broom, 1994).

The attitudes of animal users depend upon early training, traditional practices, acquisition of knowledge from others subsequent to any training, personal experience, and general beliefs and philosophy. Training in agriculture and other animal-use businesses did not, until recently, include much information about animal welfare except where it impinged on profitability. Even diseases were often mentioned in agriculture training only in relation to effects on growth, offspring production or product quantity and quality. Today's training courses are more likely to include information about the welfare of the animals and most agricultural trade journals now cover animal welfare issues. Traditional practices are often deemed by farmers, or others who keep or use animals, to be right for the sole reason that 'this is the way that we have always done it'. Although some of these methods are the best ones to produce good welfare, others are not, and traditional methods and practices should not persist just because there is a tradition to use them.

Farmers and other animal users have to live with their families, friends and neighbours. If these people are critical of the effects on the welfare of animals of the methods used, the farmer may change these methods. In some cases, the animals are very obvious to all who pass by the farm. If a sheep or cattle farmer has many animals in her fields that are noticeably lame, there will be a considerable likelihood that someone will comment on this to the farmer. Similarly, horse establishments or zoos whose animals are lame may be criticized. People in charge of animals do not like to be thought incompetent or uncaring, so they may respond to such comments by giving the animals veterinary treatment or changing the management system to avoid lameness. If the animals are inside a building or otherwise hidden from public view, the number of people who might comment on poor welfare will be smaller and there is a greater chance that the farmer or other person responsible can persuade himself or herself that there are no significant welfare problems.

Meetings with others in the same business and reading trade magazines will tend to help animal users to arrive at common views about their various problems. A farmer, laboratory-animal technician, or zookeeper who has to reconcile himself to poor welfare in some animals will find it easier to do so with the support of others. Such influences can slow down change towards better welfare in the animals, especially if economic factors mitigate against such change.

The views of the general public are largely made known to farmers and others involved in animal usage via the media. There is frequent coverage of animal welfare issues in newspapers, on radio and on television, and this affects people's attitudes by bringing scientific knowledge about animal complexity to their attention. Farmers and some other animal users may see themselves portrayed as uncaring. Some such portrayals are unfair but others are correct and the farmer cannot hide from them by putting animals in buildings and associating only with other farmers. When public demonstrations about animal welfare issues occur, the people who use the animals need to take note of them. After legislation was passed in the UK banning the keeping of calves in small crates, on animal welfare grounds, there were demonstrations by great numbers of largely orderly and apparently normal people against the shipping of calves to EU Member States where crate-housing was still permitted. These demonstrations had a big influence on farmers and politicians alike. It is not the most vociferous people (some of whom may be rather extreme in their views) who have the greatest influence on animal users or politicians, but the moderate people who represent a groundswell of public opinion. In many surveys in Europe, animal welfare has been shown to be an important issue for the general public.

Animal Welfare Science: History and Concepts

3

3.1 The History of Animal Welfare Science

3.1.1 Before 1960

Scientists and legislators now use 'animal welfare' as a term that is a scientific concept describing a potentially measurable quality of a living animal at a particular time. There are ethical questions about what people ought to do about the welfare of the animals for which they have some responsibility. However, when investigating welfare we should separate the scientific study of animal welfare from the ethical decision making. The term 'animal welfare' was not always used as a scientific concept, and indeed there are still many people who are not aware of the modern approach to the subject, so the remainder of this section concerns the historical background of the term (see also Broom, 2011).

Animals have always had welfare but what humans know of it has become modified over time, especially recently. As explained in Chapter 2 and by Broom (2003), the general human concepts of what are and are not moral actions have probably changed little over many millennia, except that the category of individuals who are considered to deserve to be treated in a moral way has broadened greatly.

Humans have long espoused the view that they have duties to others. In some human societies, for example those where the Buddhist or Jain religions dominate, the range of living individuals considered to deserve respect has long been wide. However, in most of the world, fewer of the wide variety of animals, from worms and insects to fish and mammals, are respected. Ideas about which individuals should be the subject of moral actions (Singer, 1994) have changed as explained in Chapter 2.

Before there was accurate scientific knowledge in human societies for which there are detailed records, there were descriptions of animal functioning including their behaviour, physiology and pathology. People saw very many parallels between humans and other animals and these were described by Greeks, Mayans, Chinese and others (Sorabji, 1993). Ideas about non-human animals have included the recognition of similarities to humans in respect of what would harm them, the complexity of their body regulation systems, the existence of their emotional responses and the range of abilities that they demonstrate to control their environment (Engel and Engel, 1990). Some people placed emphasis on differences between humans and all other species, as explained by Harwood (1928). The view, often thought to have originated with Descartes in the 17th century, that non-human animals are automata with almost no similarity to humans, was used in argument by some people before Descartes' time and by many people since then. It was often convenient as a way of justifying some form of exploitation of an animal. Similar arguments were used to justify slavery and other suppression of minorities. The idea that the animals we exploit are given to us for our own purposes (an interpretation of the meaning of having dominion) is also easier to maintain if those animals can be thought of as objects or automata.

Bentham (1789) stated that the key question about animals was not can they reason, but do they suffer? Most people who have lived with or looked closely at companion or farm animals have assumed that they could do both to some extent. As Duncan (2006) has said, up to the 19th century, this view was very widespread but later there was some reluctance to hold the view because of the difficulty in measuring the suffering. However, the people looking at their own animals were making observations and deducing from these. Although some may have had rather small sample sizes, this was a scientific approach.

In the 19th century and the first half of the 20th, knowledge about biological functioning increased greatly. By the end of this time, scientific disciplines such as ethology and neuroscience started to become accepted within the scientific community. In psychology prior to 1960, much of the academic tradition was human-centred and mentalistic. It was assumed that most human and non-human function could be discovered by thinking about it or by studying anatomy. Those who wanted to find out about brain function by observing behaviour and physiological change successfully challenged this view. After this change, it became scientifically dubious to refer to mental processes unless experiments or observations could directly demonstrate them. However, valuable information about brain control of behaviour spread rapidly among scientists. This did not mean that it was widely known. The division between scientists and non-scientists, and the fear of science among those narrowly educated in non-scientific disciplines, resulted in ignorance of these biological developments among those who came to have influential positions in some parts of government and industry. There are many topics, discussed in this book, which concern failures of the majority of people to understand scientific information. Attitudes to animals and understanding of brain function have both been affected by such failures. Several erroneous ideas of 100 years ago persist today.

3.1.2 The 1960s and 1970s

Ruth Harrison's book *Animal Machines* (1964) pointed out that those involved in the animal production industry were often treating animals like inanimate machines rather than as living individuals. As a consequence of this book, in 1965 the British government set up the Brambell Committee, chaired by Professor F. Rogers Brambell, to report on the matter. One of its members was W.H. Thorpe, an ethologist at Cambridge University. Thorpe emphasized that an understanding of the biology of the animals is important and explained that animals have needs with a biological basis, including some needs to show particular behaviours, and that they would have problems if the needs were frustrated (Thorpe, 1965). This view came to be written in the Brambell Report as the 'five freedoms' (Brambell, 1965). The concept of freedom has some logical and scientific difficulties, as explained in Section 2.5 and Chapter 7. However, the Brambell Report has had a beneficial influence in many countries.

Bill Thorpe was my PhD supervisor. In 1965 he asked me to comment on some material used by the Brambell Committee. This was a tape recording of hens in different housing conditions. Thorpe asked whether it was possible to deduce anything about the welfare of the birds from the sounds that they made. At that time, these tapes did not allow this, but some deduction can now be made because of the development of animal welfare science; see the work of Zimmerman *et al.* (2003) on hen vocalizations. In the 1960s, the emphasis of discussions was on animal protection, a human activity, rather than on animal welfare. In the 1970s and early 1980s, the term 'animal welfare' was used but not defined, and not considered scientific by most scientists. Animal welfare was often confused with animal rights (see Chapter 2) and such confusion still occurs.

A development of major importance to the emerging concept of animal welfare was research by ethologists and psychologists on motivation systems. The writings of Neal Miller, Robert Hinde, David McFarland and others in the 1950s to 1980s helped ethologists to understand control systems and how animals came to take decisions (Miller, 1959; Hinde, 1970; McFarland and Sibly, 1975). A review of Broom (1981a), a book entitled *Biology of Behaviour*, pointed out that the animals described in it were presented as sophisticated decision makers in almost all aspects of what they did. This view contrasted greatly with the then widespread but subsequently discredited view of animals as automata driven by 'instinct'. Key research by Ian Duncan and David Wood-Gush (Duncan and Wood-Gush, 1971, 1972), explained the motivation of animals which were frustrated because their needs were not met. Duncan, Barry Hughes, Fred Toates and Per Jensen explained the biological basis of needs (Hughes and Duncan, 1988; Toates and Jensen, 1991).

At this time there was also work on the evolution of behaviour, including sociobiology (Wilson, 1975), many of whose proponents considered motivation to be of little interest and domestic animals to be unsuitable subjects for biological research. Some of those who worked on motivation at that time changed to applied ethology studies and particularly to animal welfare, including Marian Dawkins, Ian Duncan, David Fraser, Jan Ladewig, Lindsey Matthews, Klaus Vestergaard and Piet Wiepkema, as well as the author.

The scientific use of the term 'stress' was being questioned from the late 1960s. Its use by Hans Selye was clearly ambiguous and, as J. Mason pointed out (Mason, 1968; see further explanation by Dantzer and Mormède, 1979), to some degree erroneous. The mechanisms involving the hypothalamus in the brain and the pituitary and adrenal cortex glands (HPA) and the sympathetic nervous system and adrenal medullary gland (SAM) were presented by Selye as being general to all situations, but they are not. Some people used the term 'stress' solely to mean that there was HPA axis activity, while others used it for any stimulation. Broom suggested (1983, see also Broom and Johnson, 1993) that it should be limited to adverse or potentially adverse effects with fitness reduction as the criterion. This view was supported by Dantzer, von Holst, Moberg, Mormède and Toates, but was ignored by medical and most physiological researchers.

3.1.3   Post-1980

Another view challenged in the 1970s and 1980s was the idea that domestic animals were completely modified by man and therefore scarcely biological and not comparable with their wild equivalents. Glen McBride studied a population of feral chickens on an island off Australia (McBride *et al.*, 1969). David Wood-Gush and colleagues studied another domestic fowl population (Wood-Gush *et al.*, 1978) and later, with Alex Stolba, a group of sows kept in fields with trees (Stolba and Wood-Gush, 1989). Per Jensen, encouraged by Ingvar Ekesbo, carried out a detailed study of modern domestic pigs in woodland conditions (Jensen, 1986). Based on all of this work, most ethologists concluded that the behaviour of these farm animal breeds was scarcely distinguishable in many respects from that of their wild ancestors. Another view was that of Hemmer (1983) who reviewed data indicating that domestic animals had lower brain volume than wild members of the same species. He concluded that our farm and companion animals today have less brainpower and much less complex behaviour than their wild ancestors. This view has been subsequently found to be largely incorrect (see Chapter 4). A wide range of experimental studies on learning has shown, for example, that sheep and cows recognize many individuals and that sheep have units in their brains that make this possible (Kendrick and Baldwin, 1987; Kendrick *et al.*, 1995, 2001). Also, young cattle can show an excitement response when they learn something (Hagen and Broom, 2004), and pigs can use information from mirrors after a few hours of experience with a mirror (Broom *et al.*, 2009). The major way in which domestic animals have been changed by human selection is that they are now very different from their ancestors in having some tolerance of human proximity and an ability to breed in restricted, suboptimal situations (Price, 2002).

In the 1980s, most of the animal welfare researchers were in zoology or animal production departments in universities and research institutes. Most veterinarians were aiming to benefit the animals by trying to cure or prevent animal disease. In doing this, their objective was to improve animal welfare, although many of them were not aware of the wide range of welfare topics. Some veterinarians used their clinical knowledge to ensure that the health of animals was properly considered in evaluation of welfare. A few carried out experimental work on more general aspects of animal welfare science, for example Andrew Fraser, Ingvar Ekesbo, Henrik Simonsen, Robert Dantzer, Roger Ewbank, Barry Hughes and John Webster. Andrew Fraser was one of the founders of the Society for Veterinary Ethology (later the International Society for Applied Ethology), which is still the major scientific society for animal welfare science. He was also editor of the journal then called *Applied Animal Ethology* and now called *Applied Animal Behaviour Science*, which is the most important journal for scientific papers on animal welfare. The journal *Animal Welfare* has also been of major importance in more recent years.

A few veterinarians were involved in animal welfare research in the 1980s, as mentioned above, and the paper on assessing pain and distress in laboratory animals by Morton and Griffiths (1985) had substantial influence. However, at this time most veterinarians did not consider animal welfare as a scientific discipline that should be taught to veterinary students. Neither did they think that animal welfare research was relevant to those in practice. Many thought that only veterinarians knew about animal welfare and that almost all of welfare was treatment of or prevention of disease. Animal behaviour and brain function were thought to be of minor importance to veterinary work. These views had close parallels with the medical profession, in which those who studied behavioural or mental problems were often considered peripheral to the major tasks of human medicine. Veterinarians, medical practitioners and scientists were unwilling to refer to animal feelings (Panksepp, 2005).

Research biologists in universities did not think of the study of animal welfare as a science. They were only grudgingly aware of the concept of the 3Rs (reduce, replace and refine) during laboratory animal work presented by Russell and Burch (1959). Despite the fact that many important biological systems have the function of attempting to cope with difficulties in life, the study of welfare has not been greatly valued in the scientific world, and many biologists do not think of welfare scientists as significant contributors to science. This may be related to concern among some experimental biologists that consideration of animal welfare will impair their ability to use animals in research. This view has parallels with those farmers who do not want to acknowledge that animal welfare science exists. However, the views of farmers are changing, faster than those of research scientists, as the public demands better welfare for farm animals. As consumers, members of the public can use their selective purchasing power to change farm conditions, more than they can change the attitudes of those who use animals in experiments.

Much of the discussion about the use of animals centred until relatively recently on whether or not they should be killed. Philosophers and the public were often concerned with the ethics of killing animals for human food, human clothing, scientific research or as unwanted pets (Regan, 1990; Fraser, 2008). This is an important ethical question but it is not an animal welfare issue. The animal welfare issue is what happens before death, including how they are treated during the last part of their lives, and then the method by which they are killed. However, as Haynes (2008) points out, there is a danger in this position if it results in the ethical question of whether or not it is acceptable to kill an animal being ignored or inadequately considered.

3.2   The Origins of the Animal Welfare Concept

In the 1980s, it was accepted by most biologists and veterinarians that animals and their response systems are subject to challenges from their environment. These challenges include pathogens, tissue damage, attack or threat of attack by a conspecific or predator, other social competition, excessive stimulation resulting from information processing or attempts to do so, a lack of key stimuli such as a teat for a young mammal or social contact for a social species, and insufficient stimulation because the environment is barren. In general, humans and other animals have problems if they cannot control interactions with their environment (Mason, 1968, 1971; Weiss, 1971).

The Brambell Committee did not define 'welfare' in its report but, following some generally accepted views of the functioning of animals and also the writings of Lorca, Barry Hughes (1982) proposed that the term 'animal welfare' meant that the animal was in harmony with nature, or with its environment. This is a biologically relevant statement and a precursor of later views but it is not a usable definition. Being in harmony is a single state, so it does not allow the use of scientific measures of welfare. The key question is how much the individual is in harmony. During the 1980s, the term 'welfare' was being used more and more in science, in laws and in discussion about the effects of the treatment of laboratory, farm and companion animals, hence there was a clear need for a scientific definition.

Broom (1986) used this definition of welfare: 'the welfare of an individual is its state as regards its attempts to cope with its environment'. This was further explained in a series of publications (Broom, 1988, 1991a,b; Broom and Johnson, 1993). Equivalent words in other languages include *bien-être, bien-estar, bem estar, benessere, Wohlergehen, welzijn, velfærd* and *dobrostan*. Welfare can be measured scientifically and varies over a range from very good to very poor. Welfare will be poor if there is difficulty in coping or failure to cope; 'Coping means having control of mental and bodily stability' (Broom and

Johnson, 1993). There are various coping strategies with behavioural, physio-logical, immunological and other components that are coordinated from the brain. Feelings, such as pain, fear and the various forms of pleasure, are often part of a coping strategy and feelings are a key part of welfare. The system may operate successfully so that coping is achieved, or may be unsuccessful in that the individual is harmed. One or more coping strategies may be used to attempt to cope with a particular challenge, so a wide range of measures of welfare may be needed to assess welfare. Coping with pathology is necessary if welfare is to be good, so health is an important part of welfare (Broom, 2006b).

A key point of agreement among animal welfare scientists in the early 1990s and later has been that animal welfare is measurable and hence is a sci-entific concept (see review of the ideas of Duncan, Dawkins, Broom and others by Fraser, 2008a). Another key view of animal welfare scientists is that welfare involves mental aspects. Current research on welfare involves measurements of brain function and of its consequences for behaviour and physiology (see Chapter 8). Many animal welfare indicators give information about positive and negative feelings and others evaluate health.

The World Organisation for Animal Health (OIE, 2011) followed the Broom definition when writing about what is meant by animal welfare but added an explanation:

> Animal welfare means how an animal is coping with the conditions in which it lives. An animal is in a good state of welfare if (as indicated by scientific evidence) it is healthy, comfortable, well nourished, safe, able to express innate behaviour, and if it is not suffering from unpleasant states such as pain, fear, and distress. Good animal welfare requires disease prevention and veterinary treatment, appropriate shelter, management, nutrition, humane handling and humane slaughter/killing. Animal welfare refers to the state of the animal. The treatment that an animal receives is covered by other terms such as animal care, animal husbandry, and humane treatment.

This text reads like a committee document so has some imprecise parts in it: (i) welfare is not 'how an animal is coping' but is a state that reflects how well it is coping; (ii) the animal has to cope with its whole environment, and 'the conditions in which it lives' might not mean that to all people; and (iii) the term 'innate' would not be used by any modern animal behaviour scientist as it implies 'uninfluenced by the environment' and no behaviour is uninfluenced by the environment.

There has been some controversy about the term 'welfare' and Broom's definition has been referred to by some as a functional definition and con-trasted with the feelings-related definitions of Ian Duncan (see also Broom, 2008a). Duncan argued that welfare is wholly about feelings (Duncan and Petherick, 1991; Duncan, 1993). This view was shared by some other people but a commoner position was that of Marian Dawkins (1980, 1990), who stated that the feelings of the individual are the central issue in welfare, but other aspects such as the health of that individual are also important. At the same time, those with a medical or veterinary background sometimes presented the view that health is all, or almost all, of welfare. All of Broom's papers and books discussing the welfare definition referred to feelings as a part of welfare, but even in recent times the myth that Broom's definition is functional, rather than encompassing suffering and other feelings, has been perpetuated (e.g. Dwyer and Lawrence, 2008). The idea that feelings are completely different from other biological mechanisms when individuals are trying to cope with their environment is not biologically sound. When coping is successful and problems are absent or minor, welfare is good. Good welfare is generally associated with feelings of pleasure or contentment.

Like bad feelings such as pain or fear, good feelings are a biological mechanism, and this mechanism has evolved (Cabanac, 1992; Keeling and Jensen, 2002). As discussed at length in Chapter 5, a feeling is a brain construct, involving at least perceptual awareness, which is associated with a life regulating system, is recognizable by the individual when it recurs and may change behaviour or act as a reinforcer in learning. Suffering is also defined: suffering occurs when one or more negative feelings continue for more than a few seconds or minutes (Broom, 1998). There are problems with a definition of welfare that only refers to feelings. Feelings are just one part of an animal's repertoire of coping mechanisms. Although the brain condition that results in a feeling may have first arisen accidentally, most feelings that occur now are a result of natural selection and are adaptive. Although feelings are an important part of welfare, welfare involves more than feelings; consider the examples of an individual with a broken leg but asleep, an addict who has just taken heroin, an individual greatly affected by disease but unaware of it, or an injured individual whose pain system does not function (Broom, 1991b, 1998).

The term 'welfare', although not applicable to inanimate objects or plants, is relevant to all animals because they have an ability to detect and respond rapidly to the impacts on them of their environment, usually via the functioning of their nervous system. While some of the responses of more complex animals are controlled by sophisticated processes in their brains, those of simpler animals such as worms and snails, are also part of attempts to cope with the environment. We can assess and consider the welfare of any animal. The questions: 'should we be concerned about animal welfare?', 'what should we do about poor welfare?', 'which animals should be protected?' and 'to what degree should a particular kind of animal be protected?' are separate issues. Most people think that animals with awareness are worthy of more protection.

There remain some areas of confusion, among the public and among scientists who do not specialize in the area, about what animal welfare is. In contrast, there is a substantial degree of agreement among welfare scientists about what welfare is. Points (1) to (6) below are areas where there may be some confusion in the minds of some members of the public:

1. For some people the concepts of protection of animals and animal welfare are confused. However, the first is a human action and the second is a characteristic of an animal.

2. The ethical issues about whether or not animals should be killed for human benefit are sometimes perceived to overlap with the concept of welfare, but they do not.

3. The concept of health as a key part of welfare rather than a separate topic is misunderstood by many, including medical and veterinary specialists who may not be familiar with the meaning of welfare.

4. The evolution of animals in their natural environment has led to them having certain needs that must be met for welfare to be good, and good conditions for animals will allow them to function in a natural way, i.e. a normal biological way. However, as discussed further below, naturalness is not a component of the definition of welfare.

5. The dignity of an individual is a human concept that may be applied to non-human animals, but there is no evidence that other species have such a concept. It may be used as an argument for treating animals well but it is not a part of welfare.

6. The integrity of an animal, in the sense of its wholeness, has some biological basis and is sometimes used to criticize removal of, or change in, any part of an animal's body including its limbs, appendages, organs and genotype. The procedure of damaging integrity and its consequences may affect welfare, but integrity is not a part of welfare.

Some of these areas of confusion will become less common as knowledge of welfare and its scientific study becomes more widespread. The numbers of animal welfare scientists is increasing rapidly. The subject is now being taught to veterinary students and others in all European countries, and the number of university courses on animal welfare in Brazil increased from one to over 80 between 1992 and 2012. The diversity of animal welfare science is increasing and the expansion is likely to continue. The decision by the American Veterinary Medical Association to promote the teaching of the subject in all American veterinary schools will have a substantial effect.

Animal welfare can be affected by a wide range of factors. The effects of disease, injury and starvation are negative. However, there can be beneficial stimulation, and success in actions will have positive consequences. The effects of social interactions and housing conditions may be positive or negative. In a summary of information from animal welfare research, Fraser *et al.* (2013) list ten factors to consider in order to promote good welfare in animals in production systems. Implicit in this list is the necessity to consider scientific information about the needs of animals of the species and the background under consideration. However, it is missing from their list, so it has been put at (1) in Table 3.1. Also, the word 'natural' has been changed to 'adaptive' in (4) (see Section 3.3.5) and 'euthanasia' has been changed to 'humane killing' in (8) (see Section 10.6).

The handling of animals by people will normally have negative effects on the animals' welfare but may sometimes have positive effects. Careful handling of farm animals for short periods can lead to substantial benefits for the animals in that they are less fearful of people and less likely to show escape behaviour

Table 3.1. Factors to consider in order to promote good welfare in animals in production systems (modified after Fraser *et al.*, 2013).

1	Scientific information about the needs of animals of the species and the background under consideration.
2	How genetic selection affects animal health, behaviour and temperament.
3	How the environment influences injuries and the transmission of diseases and parasites.
4	How the environment affects resting, movement and the performance of adaptive behaviour.
5	The management of groups to minimize conflict and allow positive social contact.
6	The effects of air quality, temperature and humidity on animal health and comfort.
7	Ensuring access to feed and water suited to the animals' needs and adaptations.
8	Prevention and control of disease and parasites, with humane killing if this is not feasible or recovery is unlikely.
9	Prevention and management of pain.
10	Creation of positive human–animal relationships.
11	Ensuring adequate skill and knowledge among animal handlers.

when approached and hence risk being harshly treated by people who are trying to move them. Of course, deliberate or accidental ill-treatment has negative consequences, as do most experimental procedures in laboratories and the various mutilations carried out on farm and companion animals. However, a mutilation such as the castration of a dog may have the long-term result that the individual is given much more freedom of movement than it would get if not castrated. An animal's first experience of transport is likely to induce fear and other negative effects, but after much experience of transport, the effect may be neutral or even positive. Veterinary treatment will usually have some negative short-term consequences but positive effects on welfare in the longer term. When animals are genetically changed by conventional or other breeding, the impact on the welfare of the changed animals may be neutral, negative, or positive. All the positive and negative effects on welfare, short term or long term, can be assessed scientifically using appropriate measures (Chapter 8).

The assessment of feelings is a major aim for welfare scientists (Dawkins, 1993; Broom, 1998, 2010a; Panksepp, 1998; Mendl and Paul, 2004; Paul *et al.*, 2005) and is discussed further in Chapter 8. One recent and significant development in animal welfare science has been the substantial increase in attempts to assess good welfare in a scientific way. This has become feasible because of increased acceptance of the validity of measuring positive feelings in animals. Studies such as those of Boissy *et al.* (2007) and Mendl *et al.* (2009) are increasing our understanding of animal welfare and pointing to new methods in the future.

In addition to the assessment of welfare by animal welfare scientists, it is possible to measure welfare on farm or in other places where animals are used.

Welfare outcome indicators that can be used by veterinary inspectors, farmers and others have now been worked out with considerable precision (Welfare Quality, 2009a,b,c; EFSA, 2012). It is likely that further progress will be made with measures of pain and other aspects of welfare for use by animal welfare scientists. Assessments are now being made of the risk of poor welfare and the probability of benefits to welfare (Smulders and Algers, 2009; EFSA, 2012).

3.3   Welfare in Relation to Other Concepts

3.3.1   Adaptation and welfare

The term 'adaptation' is used in an evolutionary sense and also to refer to what individuals can do (Broom, 2006a). In this latter sense, the capacity for adaptation is clearly relevant to welfare. How well can our companion, farm and laboratory animals adapt to the conditions that we impose upon them? Can wild animals adapt to our impact on them? Broom (2006a) writes: 'When referring to individual animals, adaptation is the use of regulatory systems, with their behavioural and physiological components, to help an individual to cope with its environmental conditions'. Animals can adapt better if their needs are met. What are the limits to adaptation? The idea that there are limits has been widely accepted in biology (Mount, 1979; Moberg, 1985; Beilharz, 1985) but resisted by some involved in animal production. An individual attempting to cope may fail to do so. For example, it may be difficult or impossible to cope with extreme external temperature, pathogen multiplication, high predation risk or difficult social conditions. Body state may be displaced to outside the tolerable range and death may follow. An individual may adapt to an environmental situation with difficulty, in which case the welfare is poor: for example, if an individual is adapting, or has adapted, but is in pain or depressed. Coping usually means that all mental and bodily systems have functioned so that the environmental impact is nullified. Hence 'to cope' is more than 'to adapt'. The definition of welfare refers to attempts to cope, and good welfare implies that coping is successful and is generally associated with positive feelings. However, adaptation does not necessarily mean good welfare.

3.3.2   Stress in relation to welfare

For most people, stress implies the effects of a challenge to the individual that disrupts homeostasis resulting in adverse effects. It is not just a stimulus that activates energy-releasing control mechanisms (see Section 5.2). Stimuli whose effects are beneficial would not be called stressors by most people. Also, for most people, situations that activate the hypothalamic–pituitary–adrenal cortical axis as part of a brief emergency response, but whose effects are useful to the individual, would not be called stressors. A definition of stress that is in line with the general public usage of the word is: 'stress is an environmental effect on an individual which overtaxes its control systems and results in adverse consequences, eventually reduced fitness' (Broom and Johnson, 1993, following Broom, 1983). There is no good stress, and effects that are called good stress should be called stimulation. During the development of individuals, stimuli that result from situations that are somewhat difficult for that individual can be useful experience but these are best not referred to as being stressful.

There is a clear relationship between stress and welfare in that, whenever there is stress, welfare will be poor. However, welfare could be temporarily poor, although without any long-lasting adverse effect, so without stress.

3.3.3   Needs and welfare

The needs that animals have are mechanisms that facilitate adaptation to their environment (see Chapter 7). A need is a requirement, which is part of the basic biology of an animal, to obtain a particular resource or respond to a particular environmental or bodily stimulus (Broom and Johnson, 1993). Legislation about the treatment of animals often refers to the needs of animals and it is widely accepted that welfare can only be good if the needs of the animals are met.

3.3.4   Health in relation to welfare

Health refers to what is happening in body systems, including those in the brain, which combat pathogens, tissue damage or physiological disorder. Broom (2000, 2006b) has written that 'Health is the state of an individual as regards its attempts to cope with pathology'. With disease challenge, as well as with other challenges, difficult or inadequate adaptation results in poor welfare. Health is an important part of welfare but welfare is the wider term. Conditions such as osteoarthritis in cats and dogs and sole ulcer in cows have clinical signs that are used by veterinarians in diagnosis and in the monitoring of the effects of treatment. The pain and malaise caused by the disease are components of the effects on the welfare of the animals, as are other consequences such as the disturbing effects of difficulty in locomotion and of reduced ability to obtain resources, especially in competitive situations. Indicators of poor welfare associated with disease are discussed further in Chapter 8.

The World Health Organization's definition of health since 1948 is: 'Health is a state of complete physical, mental and social well-being and not merely the absence of disease or infirmity' (WHO, 1948). I find this to be an inadequate definition because: (i) it implies that health refers to every aspect of life while I would limit health to being concerned with pathology; (ii) health is a continuum from positive to negative and the WHO definition does not allow the normal usage of the term 'poor health'; and (iii) it is difficult to differentiate welfare and health using this definition.

3.3.5   Naturalness and welfare

Where does naturalness fit with the concept of welfare? Fraser (1999) pointed out that when members of the public talk about animal welfare, their ideas often include the functioning of the animals, the feelings of the animals and the naturalness of the environment. The feelings, referred to by Fraser and others, fit comfortably into Broom's definition of welfare as they are important components of coping mechanisms and of biological functioning. Rollin (1989, 1995) advocated that 'animals should be able to lead reasonably natural lives'. This view has been reiterated by Fraser *et al.* (1997) and Fraser (2008), and in all four publications the authors refer to the importance of understanding animal needs. These authors did not say that naturalness contributes to a definition of welfare or should be part of welfare assessment. The state of an individual trying to cope with its environment will necessarily depend upon its biological functioning or, put another way, upon its nature. Natural conditions have affected the needs of the animal and the evolution of coping mechanisms in the species. The environment provided should fulfil the needs of the animal but does not have to be the same as the environment in the wild.

3.3.6   Welfare and well-being

For animal welfare scientists, the term 'welfare' refers to the positive and the negative. However, some people think only of the positive when they use the term. Well-being is generally synonymous with welfare but a higher proportion of people think just of the positive when they use it. Since welfare has been defined for many years and is the term used by most scientists and legislators, it is now considered to be the more precise term. In the USA there was initial reluctance to use 'welfare' as a scientific term because many people thought of welfare as indicating handouts to the poor. Its use by more and more scientists and by the American Veterinary Medical Association now reflects the international use of 'welfare', rather than 'well-being'.

3.3.7   Quality of life in relation to welfare

The term 'quality of life' is principally used to refer to people or companion animals who are ill or recovering from illness. In judging quality of life, the impact on the functioning of the individual, including physiological and behavioural responses and especially indicators of pain or other suffering, should be evaluated. As explained in detail in Chapter 8, the measures of welfare include all of the measures of quality of life. Both quality of life and welfare can be positive or negative, good or poor. There is some difference in the use of the terms as it would not be normal to talk about quality of life over a very short timescale such as a few hours or days. Welfare, on the other hand, can refer to short-term situations. 'Quality of life means welfare during a period of more than a few days' (Broom, 2007b). Hence quality of life can be assessed using the wide range of indicators that are available for assessing welfare.

3.3.8   Welfare and 'a life worth living'

The concept of 'a life worth living' is ethical rather than scientific, although the ethical judgements would be based on scientific information. Worth depends on a concept of value and raises the question of who decides when it is worth living or not worth living. If the individual under consideration is non-human, it is a human evaluation rather than an evaluation by the subject. This is a problem with the term 'a life worth living'. Investigation of welfare refers to a measureable quality of the animal and this is assessed in an objective way, trying to take account of what that animal needs and its current state in relation to those needs. A decision about whether or not life is worth living might not be made in the same way by the person judging and by the animal itself. A person might judge that a pet animal is in pain and that its life is not worth living. However, animals in pain still strive to survive and carry out assessments of risks to themselves. Would the animal choose to live or die? There are few reports of suicide in non-humans and most of these could have an alternative explanation. An injured prey animal, such as a goat on a mountain ledge, will only jump off the ledge when it is approached by a leopard if the risk of so doing is less than that posed by the approaching predator. If the goat did jump and died, this would be a failure of risk and benefit assessment rather than a deliberate action. The idea of a life worth living may be useful in order to criticize some housing systems or procedures on animals; but when systems or procedures are evaluated, objective measurement of welfare should be carried out on all occasions, so that the worth of the life can be properly considered.

3.4   Welfare in Relation to Sentience

Every kind of living animal makes attempts to cope with its environment. Even relatively simple animals, such as protozoans or flatworms, respond to adverse conditions such as temperatures that are too high or too low, or contact with a detectable toxic or damaging substance. The response will often be behavioural avoidance but may also be physiological change. Animals also cope with their environment by approaching or staying in areas where food or a potential mate are identified; here, they are showing positive responses to the environmental variable. In these situations, or where animals mount immunological responses to pathogens or healing responses when tissue is damaged, they are attempting to cope with their environments. Hence it is possible to consider the welfare of any animal. Animals that are sentient have the capability to use more elaborate and complex coping responses. Those animals that can have one of the higher levels of awareness and can have positive and negative feelings can use these mechanisms in order to more closely control their daily lives.

The view that we can consider the welfare of all animals, whether or not they are sentient, is not shared by all scientists. For example, Kirkwood (2006) argues that welfare is a characteristic of only sentient beings. He equates sentience with having feelings and limits the term 'welfare' to those animals that can have feelings. For arguments relating to this see Section 3.2.

While we can talk about and evaluate the welfare of any animal, people are usually more concerned about the more complex animals and may wish to protect sentient animals to a greater degree than they wish to protect animals that are not sentient. The question of how much protection should be afforded to different animals is discussed further in Chapter 10.

Brain Complexity
and Cognitive Ability

4

4.1 Brain Function and Brain Size

Although people are familiar with what a human brain is, the term 'brain' requires some explanation, since a wide range of animal species is considered here. A brain is an aggregation of nervous tissue in which some transfer and analysis of information and integration with motor output can occur. Other aggregations of nervous tissue in various parts of the body are called ganglia but the brain is normally the most complex of such aggregations in the individual. There is variation among animal groups regarding which parts of the brain have the largest volume, the most cells and the most information processing.

Some of those who have sought to compare the cognitive abilities of animals of different species have reported on total brain size, or on the size of some part of the brain (Jerison, 1973; Hemmer, 1983). While some relationships between brain size and ability have been described, larger animals generally have larger brains than smaller animals but do not have commensurate increases in intellectual ability. There are many examples of comparisons of brains where the smaller animal does not have fewer neurons. For example, one salamander species has 240,000 neurons, while a honeybee has 960,000.

The ratio between brain size and body size explains ability better than the brain size, but the relationship is far from a general one. Some animal species function very well with small brains, and some people with a small cerebral cortex can do so much of what other people can do, that the reduced cerebral cortex is not apparent in daily life. Some of these people have great intellectual ability. It is clear that the brain can compensate for lack of tissue or, to some extent, for loss of tissue. Attempts to relate ability and brain size include many anomalies so that few comparative conclusions can be reached (Barton and Dunbar, 1997; Broom, 2003). An example of a comparison that did yield an interesting result is that within the mammal orders Insectivora, Carnivora and Primates the neocortex size (expressed as a ratio to total brain size) is proportional to the size of the social group in which the animals live (Dunbar, 2000). Studies of the complexity of brain function are the way forward as these can give much information about ability as well as about welfare (Broom and Zanella, 2004).

4.2 Biology, Brain Function, Brain Structure and Cognitive Ability

Where there is reference to the brain of animals in discussions of their complexity, there has sometimes been an overt or implicit assumption that nearness in structure to humans is the best estimate of sophistication. Since humans are primates and most primates live in social groups, it is often assumed that primates have qualitatively different brain function from other animals. While primate brain function is impressive, even those whose principal work is the study of primates argue that primates do not have unique abilities, and hence are unlikely to have unique brain mechanisms (Byrne and Bates, 2007, 2010). When uniquely primate cognition is listed (e.g. Tomasello, 2000), there is often subsequent work on other species such as dogs, pigs, corvids and parrots that demonstrates lack of such uniqueness.

Estimates of brain sophistication should take account of function rather than anatomy alone because animals vary in the parts of the brain that have complex analytical functions. Although some mammals have high-level analysis functions in the cerebral cortex, a comparable high level of analysis occurs in areas of the striatum in birds and in a variety of brain regions in fish, cephalopods and other animal groups. When focusing on humans we may also over-emphasize visual analysis. Other senses have a more primary role in the lives of many mammals, fish and invertebrates. For example, although in many bird species and some mammal species the visual aspects of their world are just as important as in humans, the world of most mammals is much more olfactory than visual. The evolutionary origins of humans and other mammals, via amphibians and reptiles, is one of the many groups of fish and all on this evolutionary line are typified by expansion of the area of the forebrain that originally analysed olfactory information. Our largest brain expansion is in the cerebrum because this was the region that served that function. There is nothing unique about this part of the brain and the major expansions of the brains of some other fish are centred around the optic lobes, or the areas processing information from the lateral line organs, measuring localized pressure changes, or electro-receptors monitoring changes in patterns in the surrounding electrical field. There is substantial variation in which senses are the most important within each animal group; for example, among birds, the petrels use odour for discriminating kin from non-kin (Bonadonna and Sanz Aguilar, 2012). If we are evaluating the extent of awareness in animals or attempting to ensure that their welfare is good, we should take account of the world as they perceive it.

Humans tend to have an anthropocentric view of what is the best brain to have. It is energetically expensive to have a large brain because brain metabolism uses much energy. This means that evolutionary investment in having a large brain comes at a cost (Byrne and Bates, 2007). Animals that live a largely sedentary life often have smaller brains and less complex processing than those that have to be active and respond to many potential opportunities and dangers. For example sea squirts, which are active as larvae but as adults are attached to a solid object, have smaller brains when adult. The sedentary animal is better adapted to its environment if it has a less complex brain.

It is often thought that being a herbivore is less demanding of brainpower than being a carnivore. However, food finding, food selection and dietary balancing is often more demanding for herbivores. Also, evading predators can require more brainpower than catching prey. As a consequence, large mammalian herbivores are generally found to have more cognitive ability than large mammalian carnivores (see Section 4.4). The way of life that seems to have the greatest influence on cognitive ability and brain complexity is social living. Evaluating and responding to all of the members of social groups requires more cognitive ability, and hence brainpower, than living a solitary life (Jolly, 1966; Broom, 1981a; Humphrey, 1986, 1992). It seems that, within any taxonomic group of animals, social living is the factor most likely to lead to the evolution of an elaborate brain. Indeed, socially living animals such as the smaller squid species have much smaller brains than mammals, but have substantial abilities (Broom, 2003, 2013; Mather, 2013).

Fish brains are much more diverse in structure than those of birds or mammals but the basic plan is the same. Many of the differences in the size of the various parts of the fish brain are attributable to the sense that is most important to the group of fish. However, there has been an increase in complexity in processing ability in all of the fish groups. The complex analysis occurs in different brain regions in different fish groups. The line that led to mammals is just one of those groups so it is not surprising that the anatomical area in which the major processing occurs is not the same in mammals as in some of the other fish groups. The key question concerns the complexity of learning, cognition and emotional responses that can occur in each fish or other animal. Bshary *et al.* (2002) found that almost all abilities reported for primates can also be found in fish.

The brain of cephalopods, such as octopus and squid, is large relative to body size but is anatomically very different from that of vertebrates (Hanlon and Messenger, 1996; Broom, 2007a; Mather, 2013). The brains of other invertebrates are small in total size but not always in proportion to body size, and some have many small cells in them, so a substantial potential for complexity. The remarkable cognitive ability of some spiders is achieved with a small brain but the processing speed during evaluation of complex situations is slower than it would be in a vertebrate brain. On the other hand, the speed of life and decision making in small animals is greater than that of larger animals such as humans. As explained in Section 10.2, the fastest evaluation and responding described by Healy *et al.* (2013), who looked at humans and many other animals, was that of a blowfly.

4.3   Learning

Learning is one of the ways in which animals are affected by their environment. One definition (Broom and Johnson, 1993) is: 'learning is a change in the brain, which results in behaviour being modified for longer than a few seconds, as a consequence of information from outside the brain'. What kinds and complexities of learning are possible for the great diversity of animal taxa, and how is learning used? For any animal we can ask whether the members of the species can discriminate individuals and remember their social qualities. Also, can they learn about food, feeding places, danger in general, localized risks and other important environmental variables?

Animals are more likely to be considered sentient if they can learn much, learn fast and make few errors once they have learned (Broom, 2007a). Classical conditioning and operant conditioning can occur in animals with relatively simple nervous systems, such as the mollusc *Aplysia* (Lorenzetti *et al.*, 2006). A headless locust can learn aversive foot-shock conditioning (Carew and Sahley, 1986). Learning is not, in itself, evidence for awareness but is an indicator that further investigation of cognitive ability might reveal the existence of awareness commensurate with sentience. Comparative studies of learning ability are not easy to conduct, because learning situations usually require that an action be performed, and animals may vary in their physical ability to carry out the action.

Behavioural scientists started to compare learning ability using operants. These are actions (such as lever-pressing) carried out by an individual, with consequent effects on its environment; they are studied in a situation controlled by an experimenter. In the comparative studies, some of these operants depended upon motor abilities that were easy for some species but were very difficult or impossible for other species: for example, using a hoof to press a lever. Hence no unbiased comparison of learning ability was possible. A set of

studies by Kilgour (1987) largely overcame this problem by the use of modified Hebb–Williams mazes for animals of different sizes. These mazes start with
a decision point where there are two or more possible directions to take, one
being towards a concealed target reached after two further turns. Such a maze
still has some bias, as a comparison of learning ability: animals that often have
to navigate around their surroundings would have had more experience of a
sequence of decisions about which way to turn. This might favour animals that
use discrete pathways. However, individuals of all of the species tested have
to do this to some extent, and the locomotion required to respond in a maze
is common to all. When the numbers of errors were measured, cows, sheep,
goats and pigs performed less well than 5-year-old children but better than
dogs, cats, rats, horses and several other mammals and birds. When speed of
learning was compared in the same study, the sequence was very similar, but
dogs performed as well as the farm ungulates.

4.4   Discrimination and Recognition

It might be expected that social animals, for example cows, pigs and dogs,
would be able to recognize individuals of their own or of other species. The
first step in investigating this question is to attempt to establish whether or
not they can discriminate between individuals. Discrimination might occur
without recognition. Recognition involves distinguishing among individuals and then using the information to facilitate social interaction. Pigs
(Mendl *et al.*, 2002; McLeman *et al.*, 2005) and dogs (Sommerville *et al.*,
1993) are among the species that have been shown to be able to discriminate between and respond to conspecifics and other animals using olfac-
tion. Cattle have been trained to go towards one conspecific rather than
another in order to get a food reward (Hagen and Broom, 2003). In a series
of studies with sheep, Kendrick and colleagues demonstrated behavioural
discrimination of individual sheep and humans and identified neurons in
the medial temporal and prefrontal lobes of the cerebral cortex that fired
only when particular individuals were seen. These discriminations of pairs
of photographs could still be shown and the specific cells could still be found
1–2 years after the training period, so sheep memory is long (Kendrick
and Baldwin, 1987; Kendrick *et al.*, 1995, 2001). When a ewe recognizes
her lamb between 2 and 12 h after birth, changes in the brain are associated with the behavioural process. Certain brain changes started after
2 h and were consolidated over a 10-h period. Production of brain-derived
neurotrophic factor and its receptor trk-B occurred at 4–5 h after birth,
and there was messenger RNA expression in the olfactory and visual processing systems, temporal cortex, four other cortical regions, hippocampus
and amygdala (Broad *et al.*, 2002).

   A further level of recognition, perhaps involving some similar mechanisms, is to distinguish individual state and respond to it physiologically and

behaviourally. Elliker (2007) trained sheep to approach photographs of sheep with a calm expression rather than those of sheep with a startled expression, or vice versa. Elliker also found, using computer-modified photographs, that the ear position was the main feature used by the sheep to make this distinction, rather than eye features.

4.5   Cognition

Cognition was defined by Shettleworth (1998, 2010) as 'the mechanisms by which animals acquire, process, store and act on information from the environment'. Many authors including Mendl and Paul (2004) and Paul *et al.* (2005) refer to Shettleworth's definition of cognition. However, a high proportion of all brain function is included within this definition: for example, some perceptions and motor system outputs would be included, but these would not normally be considered as part of cognition. The basis of Shettleworth's definition is that during cognition something is formed in the brain that represents what is acquired and processed and can be retained and subsequently used. In a summary of what is included in cognition, Heyes (2000) included:

1. an entity in the brain;
2. 'input from other cognitive states and processes and from perception'; and
3. 'outputs to other cognitive states and processes and to behaviour'.

A key aspect of cognition is that the entity in the brain does not disappear when perception ceases. Hence Terrace (1984) argued that cognition involves explicit representations of absent stimuli. This is an insufficient definition by itself because the representation would often be of more than just stimuli and would itself be a result of processing inputs in relation to other relevant information. A definition proposed here is: cognition is having a representation in the brain of an object, event or process, in relation to its context, where the representation can exist whether or not the object, event or process is directly detectable or actually occurring at the time. The representation of something absent is an abstraction.

Our understanding of cognitive ability in humans and other animals is based on our own observations of behaviour during the course of everyday life, on those reported to us by people whom we know or hear about and on the results of experimental studies conducted with the purpose of improving that understanding. As mentioned above, social interactions are among the most demanding intellectual challenges encountered, so some conclusions about cognitive ability are deduced as a consequence of observing these. Learning in social situations has been described for many species of animals (Box and Gibson, 1999). In the course of such studies, there may be different responses to different individuals and actions indicating awareness of intentions and of social strategies. An attempt to categorize these strategies was the division into active or passive, otherwise described as proactive or reactive (Koolhaas *et al.*, 1999). However, based on such evidence, it is not easy to write about the concepts that the animals are likely to have. There are many descriptions of the behaviour of social animals, and of some of the cognitive functioning deduced to be associated with it. The ethologist studying social and other behaviour may accept without question that animals of a species have a certain level of cognitive ability. However, evidence from experimental studies is required by some other biological scientists before they accept that the cognition occurs. There is much evidence about cognitive ability as a result of observation of animals in free-moving situations. However, it is important that there should be refinements in precision of observation and the development of field experiments so that valid and convincing information about the ability can be obtained. Anecdotal or unsubstantiated information suggesting certain levels of cognitive ability need further investigation (Hauser, 2000).

4.6   Range of Cognitive Abilities

In this section, examples of studies indicating various degrees of cognitive ability are presented. The implications for awareness, in some cases with reference to these studies, are discussed in Chapter 6.

As a result of learning, all animals consolidate memories and acquire knowledge; that is, information that can be used subsequently. Most gain expertize, in that they become more accomplished at tasks. Sometimes it is apparent to the human observer that the individual is deliberately practising a movement and relating the actions to perceived input resulting from them (Helton, 2005). Spiders can build a web without having done so before but their web structure and choice of location improve with practice. This raises the (as yet unanswered) question of whether or not the spider has a concept of the web before it is built. We can ask the same question about human activities. A young child can make crawling movements without having done so before, but locomotion improves with practice. During the practice, very many sensory inputs are received that are a result of the child's muscle usage. While some components of the child's locomotion are, or become, largely automatic, other components are susceptible to modification according to the sensory inputs received. The child may have a concept of stimuli that might alter these components. In the same way, spiders might have concepts of the likely consequences of those components of web-building that may be altered if certain stimuli are received. It is not possible to state categorically that spiders do not have such concepts and, as research on cognition in jumping spiders progresses, the likelihood that the spiders have such concepts increases.

Which animals have cognitive representations of objects or other resources? At one time it was thought that a chicken would lose any concept of an object if it were out of sight. However, studies by Vallortigara and colleagues showed that not only could young domestic chicks go to objects hidden behind screens, but that when two or three objects were hidden behind screens, the chicks went to the screen with the larger number of objects (Rugani *et al.*, 2009).

Other experimental studies show that domestic animals can use a visual or auditory symbol for objects. Langbein *et al.* (2004) were able to train goats to respond by carrying out an operant in order to get water when they saw one particular picture rather than others. A second example is familiar to those who have trained dogs, but it has been studied in one female dog in a carefully controlled way by Rossi and Ades (2008). When a dog was given commands that required her to respond to one of several objects, such as a ball, a stick, a bottle, a key or a toy bear, and to carry out one of several actions, such as point to it or fetch it, she was successful. Similarly, Kaminski *et al.* (2009) found that dogs shown replicas or photographs could use this information and fetch the objects that were thus iconically portrayed. When Rossi and Ades' dog was provided with a keyboard that had symbols on it indicating 'water', 'food', 'stroke me', 'I go out', 'I get a toy', or 'I urinate', she could indicate what she detected or what she wanted to do next. A further example is of pigs studied by Held *et al.* (2000). They were put in a room and allowed to find hidden food. On the next day they were returned to the room and went immediately to the place where they had found food. These studies show that some of these animals had a concept of an object in the absence of that object, had a concept of a symbol or of a location and had a concept that pressing the symbol or going to a particular place was linked in a causal way to obtaining the resource. For a review of pig cognition see Held *et al.* (2002).

Whenever individuals move from one place to another they have some potential to learn routes. Subsequent to taking a route, the individual may have a concept of the route taken. Van Schaik *et al.* (2013) have described how orang-utans plan routes and communicate plans to others. A high proportion of the abilities described for the orang-utans have also been described in bees, ants, and various fish and birds.

Copying the actions of others requires a significant level of cognitive ability. However, when experiments are carried out to assess this, the nature of the action to be copied in relation to motor ability will result in some actions being easy for an animal and some being difficult, so this has to be taken into account when evaluating the information given about awareness. When the bonobo Kanzi was trained to use words, this was done with the use of a lexigram keyboard. Kanzi not only learned to use lexigrams but also to understand and respond to several hundred spoken English words. When asked to take or do something, using 660 novel sentences such as 'give Karen a carrot', 'make the dog bite the snake' or 'make the snake bite the dog', Kanzi did the correct thing for 81% of the sentences (Rumbaugh *et al.*, 2000).

Some birds, for example many parrot species and song birds, have very good ability to copy the vocalizations of others. Among the most impressive demonstrations of the awareness and cognitive ability are those of an African grey parrot (*Psittacus erithacus*) (Pepperberg, 2000). The parrot was trained to respond to various objects and to use words. He learned to name each object correctly. He also said the correct words for seven colours, five different shapes and quantities from one to six. Requests to be given particular objects or to be able to carry out certain actions were also made by the parrot. Humans find the ability to use words in context particularly impressive, but many animals cannot impress in this way because they cannot make the appropriate sounds, and we cannot recognize any other kinds of 'words' that they produce.

In some cases, animals have to learn that immediately detectable information about the location of a resource has to be modified in a specific way in order that the resource can be obtained. One example, for animals of several species, is to make a detour around a fence in order to get to a resource. This has been shown for chickens (Regolin *et al.*, 1995); for dogs (Pongrácz *et al.* (2005); and for other species, including tortoises (*Geochelone*), provided they have watched another tortoise do it (Wilkinson *et al.*, 2010).

Another well-known example of an animal carrying out an action in the absence of the agent enforcing that action is a trained individual performing when alone. Dogs will keep doing what they have been encouraged or trained to do by humans when the human is not present. Performance occurs in some circumstances but not in others, for example terrorized or sulking dogs may not perform (Coppinger and Coppinger, 2001).

If an individual has the novel visual experience of viewing images in a mirror, this could be followed by learning about what it sees in the mirror in relation to itself and then using such information at a later time. Human infants can use mirrors in the course of shape discrimination (Itakura and Imamizu, 1994) and, if given sufficient exposure to mirrors at appropriate age, will discover the contingency between visual and proprioceptive feedback from their own body movements (Lewis and Brooks-Guy, 1979). At 5 months of age they look more at their own image in a mirror than at the image of another infant or a puppet (Bahnick *et al.*, 1996) and at 9 months they are able to discriminate self from other in a mirror (Rochat and Striano, 2002). When looking in a mirror at 14–18 months, infants are described as showing self-referencing activities, self-labelling and embarrassment at rouge on the face (Bertenthal and Fisher, 1987). These children would have been told that the image in the mirror was of themselves. Povinelli *et al.* (1996) allowed children to see a television image of themselves that was very similar to a mirror image, and found that when a sticker was put on their heads, no 2-year-olds reached for the sticker, 25% of 3-year-olds reached for it and 75% of 4-year-olds reached for it.

Menzel *et al.* (1985) also used live television images and reported that chimpanzees could use these images to find targets visible only on the television screen. Iriki *et al.* (2001) observed that Japanese monkeys could use televised images of their hands to pick up food, while capuchin monkeys were shown live television images of themselves in research by Anderson *et al.* (2009). The authors concluded that their behaviour strongly suggested recognition of the correspondence between kinaesthetic information and external visual effects. Dolphins have been reported to use a television image, apparently to explore themselves visually (Marten and Psakoros, 1995). Tests with chimpanzees, an elephant, dolphins and magpies with previous experience of mirrors, using marks on the body visible in a mirror, led to the individuals touching or apparently looking at the marks (Gallup, 1982, 2002; Reiss and Marino, 2001; Plotnik *et al.*, 2006; Prior *et al.*, 2008).

Broom *et al.* (2009) exposed 4–6-week-old pigs to a mirror for the first time in such a way that they could see a food bowl otherwise out of view behind a barrier (Fig. 4.1). The young pigs went behind the mirror to the apparent position of the food bowl. However, when given 5 h experience of a mirror, they responded initially to it as if to another pig. Later they looked at it as they moved and then stood still, apparently looking at their image and its surroundings, oriented either with nose towards the mirror or with the head parallel to it. Because of the lateral position of the pig's eye, it is not possible to record duration of looks towards the mirror, and pigs show little change in facial expression. Some pigs vocalized. As with the movements in front of a novel mirror described for chimpanzees, humans, capuchin monkeys, dolphins and elephants (Gallup, 1982; Reiss and Marino, 2001; Keenan *et al.*, 2003; Plotnik *et al.*, 2006; Anderson *et al.*, 2009) some of the movements of these young pigs suggest that they could have been monitoring the movements in the mirror image when they moved their own head or body (Fig. 4.2). After this experience with the mirror, seven out of eight pigs tested in the apparatus in Fig 4.1 moved away from the mirror and around the barrier to the food bowl. Location by odour was prevented by fans and the naïve controls had exactly the same olfactory situation. To use information from a mirror and find a food bowl, each pig must have: (i) observed features of its surroundings; (ii) remembered these and its own actions; (iii) deduced relationships among those observed, remembered features; and (iv) acted accordingly.

The abilities indicated by these mirror and television image studies range from discrimination of images, through learning that what is seen in a mirror is on the same side as the observer, learning that one's own movements can be monitored by looking at the mirror, to appreciating that the image is the self. As Rochat (2002) puts it, in this last case the image is standing for the identified or conceptual self, not somebody else, and the self is as seen by others. The significance of mirror studies in relation to awareness and the issue of self-awareness is discussed further in Section 6.6.

The discrimination of how many objects are present is widely reported in mammals and birds for small numbers of objects. A study by Agrillo *et al.* (2009) showed that mosquito-fish could learn to differentiate between two and three symbols on a card, and Reznikova (2007) reported discrimination between different numbers of objects by ants. The ability to count up to eight has been demonstrated in several non-human animals. Among the most impressive recent studies on counting is the work of Anna Smirnova in Moscow (personal communication, 2013) who has trained hooded crows to respond to collections of one to eight dots and written numbers from 1 to 8. The crows could also add two sets of dots totalling up to eight, and two written numbers totalling up to 8.

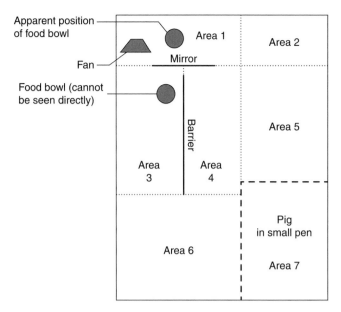

Fig. 4.1. Plan of the pen where the experiments were carried out, showing the small pen with solid walls (Area 7), mirror in a frame, solid wood barrier, fan position (above pig head level in the pen, to prevent detection by odour) and the numbers of floor sections used to describe the position of the pig. Area 3 is where the red food bowl, whose reflection was visible in the mirror when the pig was in Areas 4 or 7, was placed during the mirror test. The food bowl would appear to be in Area 1 to a naïve pig that had not had experience with a mirror. The pig had not been given food in this place before the experiment.

Time estimation is evident from many animal learning studies. Rosati *et al.* (2007) found that chimpanzees would choose to wait extra minutes in order to get a larger food reward, rather than an immediate smaller reward. The impressive work of Clayton and collaborators on jays and other members of the crow family (e.g. Raby and Clayton, 2009) is described in Chapter 6.

Cognitive ability and awareness in fish is discussed by Chandroo *et al.* (2004). We know that some fish must have mental representations of their environment in relation to their ability to navigate (Reese, 1989; Rodriguez *et al.*, 1994) and that they have the ability to recognize social companions (Swaney *et al.*, 2001). Fish can avoid places where they encountered a predator (Czanyi and Doka, 1993) or were caught on a hook (Beukema, 1970) for some months or years. Some fish species can learn spatial relationships and form mental maps (Odling-Smee and Braithwaite, 2003) and can use information about sequences of spatial information (Burt de Perera, 2004). The parts of the brain used to achieve this are not anatomically the same in fish (Broglio *et al.*, 2003) as in mammals but the function is very similar. It is clear that the timing of events can be integrated to allow the fish to produce appropriate avoidance

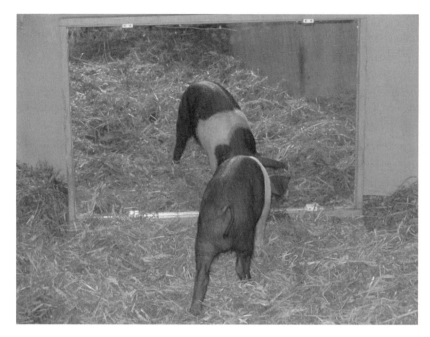

Fig. 4.2. The movements of young pigs in front of the mirror, to which the animals were exposed for 5 h, often suggested that they were looking at their image while making body movements (photograph D.M. Broom).

responses (Portavella *et al.*, 2004; Yue *et al.*, 2004) and it is difficult to explain the results of these studies without assuming that the fish feel fear. The learning ability demonstrated in a range of studies (Sovrano and Bisazza, 2003) indicates sophisticated cognitive processes more complex than associative learning. In recent years, many studies of mammals and birds have indicated that the animals may use different strategies at different times in order to cope with the same problem. When Schjolden *et al.* (2005) investigated individual variation in the responses of trout to a difficult situation, it was clear that the fish were using coping strategies involving agonistic behaviour or physiological responses, or both, to deal with the problem.

The cognitive abilities of cephalopods have been described by Mather (1995, 2013), Mather and Anderson (2007) and by Broom (2007a). Some of the evidence has been described by Nixon and Young (2003) and EFSA (2005). Cephalopod perceptual ability is substantial, as is their brain complexity. Experience affects their behaviour development and they have sophisticated learning ability with long-term and short-term memory. Cephalopods can modify previous learning, learn mazes, use flexible route-planning, have individual differences, show simultaneous different responses to individuals on the two sides of the body, use tools and carry out behaviour that leads to deception. Their ability to change colour seems to be associated with an unpleasant emotion, such as after fighting or handling. Social cuttlefish and squid show specific colour pattern changes in situations that appear to involve risk of attack and hence fear in the animals (Moynihan, 1985). Cephalopods show colour change and behavioural response to crowding and danger (Budelmann, 1998; Boal *et al.*, 1999; Messenger, 2001).

Decapod crustaceans exhibit complex learning ability and there is good evidence for memory lasting several days (Tomsic *et al.*, 1996; Feld *et al.*, 2005; Gherardi and Atema, 2005). For example, hermit crabs that compete for shells can remember which shells they have previously investigated (Jackson and Elwood, 1989). Crabs and other decapod crustaceans show avoidance learning (Elwood *et al.*, 2009). The spiny lobster *Panulirus argus* (Lohmann *et al.*, 1995) can orientate by use of a magnetic sense. If the animals were displaced for 12–37 km, they were capable of accurate orientation towards their home location. This was in the absence of visual or magnetic cues on the outward journey and of visual cues at the test site. The animals demonstrated a sense of location relative to home location using cues at the test site and must have remembered the magnetic and visual details of their home during their long journey.

Classical conditioning and operant conditioning can occur in the swimming sea slug *Aplysia* (Lorenzetti *et al.*, 2006), while context specific learning has been described in *Aplysia* and in the pond snail *Lymnaea* (Haney and Lukowiak, 2001).

Fruit flies (*Drosophila*) have been demonstrated to show associative conditioning, incidental learning, contextual learning and second-order conditioning (Greenspan and van Swinderen, 2004). Cockroaches can show place learning (Mizunami *et al.*, 1998), and both honeybees *Apis mellifera* (Menzel *et al.*, 2005) and ants (Reznikova, 2003, 2007) have been described as having the ability to form cognitive maps. This implies that information obtained at different points on a journey is gathered together in an allocentric representation; thus the individual has a concept of spatial relationships without being able to perceive cues relevant to them at the time. Reznikova also described ants learning by observation, counting while foraging and transmitting learned information to other ants. The ability of honeybees to transmit information on returning to the hive after foraging has been known for many years. The ants and the bees must be remembering information about their spatial movements when transmitting such information to others. Bees are able to discriminate patterns, generalize (e.g. sameness versus difference or symmetry versus asymmetry) and use information in a novel situation.

The jumping spider *Portia* has been shown to look at a maze, move out of sight of it and then choose the optimal route through the maze when they can only see the entry point (Tarsitano and Jackson, 1994, 1997). For further information on awareness in spiders and other animals see Jackson and Cross (2011) and Chapter 6.

4.7   Metacognition

Metacognition means to know what you know. Can non-humans have this capacity? The studies of Hampton (2001) indicate that it may be present in rhesus monkeys. Hampton presented monkeys with an image and then after a delay, four images including the original to which they had to respond to obtain a peanut, a preferred reward. After learning what would happen during the test, the monkeys were given the choice of:

1. Taking the test, with the peanut as a potential reward, and risking getting no reward if they were not correct; or
2. Not taking the test and receiving a less-preferred food item.

When this was done, the monkeys chose to try the test, if the delay between the presentation of the first image and the test was short. However, the longer the delay, the less likely it was that the monkeys would choose the test and the more likely that they would just accept the less-preferred reward. This result is interpreted as indicating that the monkeys were aware of their potential to forget the first image if the delay before the test was greater. There have been several other studies with various species indicating capacities for metacognition in humans, monkeys and dolphins but not in rats or pigeons (Smith *et al.*, 2003; Mendl and Paul, 2004). Metacognition is also involved in some of the studies discussed in Section 4.8 on innovative behaviour.

4.8   Innovation

In human society, innovation is highly regarded. Innovation is said to occur when a new solution to a problem, or an action that meets new requirements, is discovered. The innovation may be something that is new in the whole community or may just be new for the particular individual. There are many examples of innovation by non-humans being observed. These are reviewed by Reader and Laland (2003). Innovative or creative behaviour occurs spontaneously only at low frequencies so is typically missed by standardized observations of animals (Bates and Byrne, 2007). As a consequence, in order to obtain information about cognitive abilities of animals, anecdotal evidence may have to be used. Bates and Byrne proposed that anecdotal observations can be used if: (i) they are by observers experienced with the species; (ii) the records were originally recorded in detail at or very soon after the observation; and (iii) there are multiple independent records of the same phenomenon. An example of this being done was an investigation of tactical deception in primates. An early observation that they described was of a young baboon that was being chased by an adult male stopping, standing on its hind legs and looking into the distance. This would be a normal reaction to seeing a predator or rival baboon troop, but the human observers using binoculars could see no source of danger to the baboon. The pursuing male was distracted from the chase and spent time looking in the same direction and the chase was not resumed. Similar cases of apparent deception have been seen in various primate species by many observers. The action by the young monkey might indicate an awareness of the way in which the chasing monkey would think, or might just be a tactic that had been accidental, and then successful, so has been learned. However, the probability of such an action arising accidentally seems very low and the likelihood that the monkey has some awareness of the mental state of the other individual seems greater (Whiten and Byrne, 1988, 1997).

In various published papers indicating that cognitive phenomena are real, Lefebre *et al.* (1997) considered 322 reports of innovations in foraging methods used by birds, and Reader and Laland (2002) considered 533 reports of innovation, 445 of social learning and 607 of tool use in primates. Both studies found that the birds or primates with a larger striatum or neocortex of the brain were more likely to show the innovative behaviour. Innovation is also reported for other vertebrates. For example, catfish were shown in a media video to come to the edge of an area of water where doves came to drink and to catch and eat the doves.

Many examples of innovative behaviour in the scientific literature report on tool use. For example, crows are reported to use a tool to get to a second tool that can be used for accessing food (Taylor *et al.*, 2007). The human preoccupation with tool use is obviously related to our own capabilities but the literature bias towards tool use should not be taken to mean that it is the most impressive cognitive ability. While tool use does require substantial ability, it is necessarily limited to animals such as primates, which have hands, and birds, which have a bill and sometimes feet with which they can pick up objects. Animals without such anatomical equipment may have cognitive ability that is just as complex. For example: (i) ten Cate and colleagues (van Heijningen *et al.*, 2013) and other researchers have investigated whether or not birds and primates can learn abstract rules; (ii) many studies have been carried out on learning sets in animals; (iii) the ability of animals to learn what can be seen in a mirror has been studied; and (iv) the extent to which individuals can learn to deceive others in order to gain resources has been investigated. Sequences of behaviour previously thought to have been largely automatic, such as nest-building in weaver birds, are now known to include flexible components and occasions when there is innovation (Walsh *et al.*, 2013).

Innovative behaviour may be transmitted within social groups. If it is, the process may later be called 'culture'. Jane Goodall (1963) observed chimpanzees in Gombe, Tanzania, using thin sticks to put into the exits from termite mounds, withdraw them and eat the termites clinging to them. She noted that the behaviour appeared to be copied by others and this might be an example of culture 'behaviour patterns transmitted by imitation or tradition'. As indicated in this description, culture includes actions and beliefs that are not innovative and may be widespread or universal in societies of the species, referred to as 'human universals' by Brown (1991). Bill McGrew (e.g. McGrew and Tutin, 1978) described culturally transmitted activities in chimpanzees such as hammering oil palm fruits, smashing baobab fruits on a branch, drumming on a wooden sounding board, using leaves as a sponge, dragging branches, using a grooming hand-clasp, and bathing in pools or entering caves during very hot weather. Similar actions have been described in bearded capuchin monkeys in Boa Vista, Brazil, and long-tailed macaque monkeys in Thailand (Gumert et al., 2009). Some of these activities are universal in the species while others have been described in only one or a few populations. As Whiten et al. (2001) emphasized, there is cultural variation in chimpanzees and other primates, as there is in humans.

A wide range of variation in behaviour, some associated with innovation, has also been described in social bird species. The work of Clayton, Emery and collaborators on jays, rooks and crows (e.g. Raby and Clayton, 2009) is described in Chapter 6. A recent observation in Israel, presented in a media video, was of crows that gathered bread but did not eat it, took it to the edge of an area of water, dropped it in the water and then caught the fish that were attracted to it. Members of the social group of crows watched such behaviour and copied it.

4.9 Cognitive Bias

When a situation is evaluated, there will often be some degree of ambiguity in the information available. In some circumstances the same sensory input could indicate that there is a likely consequence that could be either positive or negative. As Mendl et al. (2009) put it, should an individual interpret a rustle in the grass as danger or as food? This depends on the overall set of information available. In a series of studies, Mendl and collaborators have investigated the possibility that an animal's interpretation of an ambiguous situation may be altered by its emotional state, those in negative states being the more likely to respond as if the negative outcome will occur. The influence of affect on a range of cognitive processes including attention, memory and judgement has been called cognitive bias (Paul et al., 2005; Mendl et al., 2009). The bias referred to here is not a bias in the cognitive mechanism but rather in the direction of the decision reached.

Harding et al. (2004) presented rats with one tone followed by positive consequences, and another followed by negative consequences, and then tested them with an intermediate tone. Rats that had been living in a relatively rich environment were more likely to respond to an ambiguous tone as positive. Similarly, Burman et al. (2008) found that rats from a better environment treated an ambiguous food bowl position as positive. Mendl et al. (2010b) found that rescue shelter dogs with a higher separation anxiety score were more likely to react to an ambiguous position as negative. Doyle et al. (2011) trained sheep that there was a positive and a negative bucket position. If they were shown a bucket in an ambiguous position between the positive and negative positions, they did not go to it after being stressed. Studies using such a paradigm, reviewed by Mendl *et al.* (2009), had results indicating cognitive bias in 75% of cases. The fact that some cases did not indicate it requires consideration of what might influence the results of such studies.

Do the cognitive bias studies reveal affect accurately? Do they indicate how good or how poor welfare is? Key information needed in order to answer this is whether or not any non-affect factor could lead to cognitive bias. It may not be possible to know all such factors. The existence of cognitive bias may well give information about the emotional state of the animals and about their welfare, but in order to understand cognitive bias there is a need to consider the strategies adopted by individuals in life as a whole, and in the test situation. What are the possible strategies, which of these are shown, and what will be the consequences of showing one or other strategy? Once this is ascertained, the probability that the supposed optimistic or pessimistic response will be shown can be calculated and compared with the data obtained (Broom, 2010a).

Would cognitive bias generally be adaptive? It may be good for people to look for positive aspects of any situation and advantageous to be optimistic. However, an 'accurate evaluation strategy', or even a 'look hard for the negative as it may be too risky not to do so strategy' may also be effective. These strategies may also be associated with good welfare in the individuals that use them. Hence the link between an optimistic evaluation and good welfare, or between a pessimistic evaluation and poor welfare, may not always be close.

It may well be, as assumed in cognitive bias studies, that a depressed individual will interpret ambiguous signals in a negative way. However, an individual that is feeling bad, and whose welfare is poor, might still have some probability of selecting the positive option because of a degree of randomness in action, or might do so as a strategy in an attempt to achieve the positive by selecting a cue associated with the positive. An expected level of positive selections might be calculated. If a positive bias is present, does it always mean that the welfare is good? There could be a link between the condition of the animal and the actual test used. The condition of the animal, and how that condition is engendered, may be related to positive and negative emotions. Suppose that the smell of cut hay engenders a positive affect in an individual. If this individual smells it and then evaluates all slightly ambiguous situations as positive, does this mean that its welfare is good? The test may be giving information about immediate past experience rather than about welfare in the longer term. It would seem essential, in interpreting the results of cognitive bias tests, to take account of those of other tests. Data on cognitive bias are a useful addition to our repertoire of scientific studies of welfare. However, if there is additional information then the welfare evaluation will be more reliable.

In conclusion, cognitive bias is a potentially valuable indicator of affect and of welfare. However, it has not yet been demonstrated that either the affect, or the welfare, will be reliably indicated by cognitive bias studies alone.

A combination of studies is needed to increase the accuracy with which cognitive bias reveals feelings or allows assessment of welfare.

4.10   Variability Among Individuals and Within Populations

It is widely accepted by biologists in general, and by behaviour scientists in particular, that there is much variation among individual humans and among individuals of other species. The majority of this variation is a consequence of the great range of environments in which individuals develop and hence in the diversity of their experiences. A further cause of variation is a result of differences in the genetics of individuals. Although we know that there is this variation, we often refer to whole species as if all were the same. Another assumption made is that it is possible to generalize about people from a particular city or country or those who have a particular religion. Statements are also made about the behaviour and abilities of people of a certain race or dogs of a certain breed. Such generalizations will often be wrong, and are especially unlikely to be correct if they imply uniformity in the behaviour of, for example, the people from a country or dogs of a breed. The most that can be said with any accuracy is that there is a certain probability that individuals in a category will have a given characteristic.

Generalizations about the brains and behaviour of people and other animals are often made and are seldom correct. In comparisons between relatively closely related species, there is more variation within species in most cognitive abilities and emotional capacities than between species. Variable species include individuals that are much worse than average in respect of any ability. For example, a person with advanced dementia is much worse at learning than the average pig, or rat, or salmon. Hence most generalizations about cognitive ability and emotional capacities should be considered to refer to the average individual, unless further information is provided. In some cases, it is apparent that only the most able individuals within a species are being compared.

When studies of learning, cognition and emotional capacity are conducted in humans, the subjects are usually university students, or people who volunteer for such projects, or people who want to be paid to be subjects. The first two groups and many of those in the third group are likely to be more intellectually capable than the average person. There will also be biases in the selection of non-human animals for such studies. Since the experimental studies are difficult or impossible to carry out unless the subject is very tolerant of the close proximity of humans, in many species few subjects can be found. As a result, our knowledge is mainly about very tame animals. Some of the most interesting results are obtained using only one animal: for example, the African grey parrot studied extensively by Irene Pepperberg (2000). A study of one animal does tell us what is possible for a member of the species. It does not mean that all individuals have the ability.

The capabilities of individuals to respond effectively to stimuli and to cope with environmental impacts will vary. A given situation might be easy for one individual to cope with but impossible for another, apparently similar, individual to cope with. Hence, within a group exposed to a condition, welfare may be very poor in some but quite good in others. If our objective is to minimize poor welfare, we have to know about the ability to cope of the least able in the group.

4.11 Capabilities for Morality

What is needed in order to behave in a moral way? This means in a way that results in: (i) avoidance of harm to others; (ii) benefit to others; or (iii) increase in the stability of the social group. Animals need to have brain function that allows some degree of recognition, awareness, decision making and feelings in order to behave morally (Barton and Dunbar, 1997; Broom, 2006c). There must be social living for a long enough time.

Many studies of social behaviour include implied evidence for individual recognition, for example, in vervet monkeys (Cheney and Seyfarth, 1990). Experimental studies with cattle (Hagen and Broom, 2003) show that they can be trained to approach one individual rather than another in order to gain a food reward. Kendrick *et al.* (2001) found that sheep could be trained to discriminate between individual conspecifics and individual humans (see Section 4.4).

Other aspects of cognitive ability relevant to the development of moral behaviour have been demonstrated in many animals. Most of the literature on non-humans is on primates (Harcourt, 1992; Byrne, 1995; Lee, 1999; Heyes and Huber, 2000). In a study of sheep in alpine pastures, Favre (1975) found that flocks led by an old ewe would graze a pasture and then avoid revisiting it until about 30 days later, by which time it had regrown. Many non-human species would appear to be capable of some degree of awareness, as defined and categorized by Sommerville and Broom (1998), and also complex decision making and a variety of feelings (Broom, 1998). An indication of the possible awareness of own actions and functioning comes from the studies of Hagen and Broom (2004) on young cattle. The heifers were put in a pen whose gate could be opened by pressing a panel with the nose, thus giving access to food 15 m away. They learned to do this, and at the time of learning showed an excitement response of increased heart rate and jumping or galloping. This 'eureka' effect was not shown by controls, which just gained access to the reward, or by heifers which had learned earlier how to open the gate.

In order that an individual behaves in a moral way, there must be an appropriate motivational system. Motivational state is the sum of the states of a set of causal factors, and the mechanisms which give rise to these will have evolved like any other biological mechanism (Broom, 1981a). The evolution of morality will therefore depend substantially on the evolution of the motivational system. The higher brain processes that are used when using all available information to make complex decisions will be a very important aspect of the biological processes underlying morality.

The idea that there was a great change from non-human communication to human language, with an associated jump in complexity of cognitive function, is not now regarded as logical (Leavens, 2007). Examples from primates come from chimpanzees and orang-utans that modify their visual and auditory signals to humans according to the current situation and the reward context. Many other social mammals and birds have complex visual signalling systems that are comparable to aspects of human language.

4.12   The Dangers of Occam's Razor

The brains of humans and of those animals domesticated by humans are very complex and our information about brain function, while improving, is still limited. One approach to science when considering the functioning of biological systems is to apply Occam's razor or Lloyd Morgan's canon (Lloyd Morgan, 1896). These approaches require that simple explanations for phenomena should be considered first and more complex explanations used only if the simpler ones are not satisfactory. Where there are several explanations for brain systems (some simpler and some more complex), if the Occam's razor approach is used it may never be possible to justify a complex explanation. However, given the nature of the brain, it may be that the simple explanations are wrong and the complex explanations are right (Broom, 2003). Future knowledge may be needed to be completely sure of this. In these circumstances, it could be misleading, and it could slow down progress in science, to insist on accepting the simple explanation. I consider that this has happened for many years and that the development of our understanding of brain-based phenomena has been harmed by such attitudes.

Some of those who use animals for food production or sport deny complex brain functioning (including feelings) in animals, perhaps because knowledge of this might prevent aspects of the usage. It may be that some scientists use the argument requiring that simple explanations must be used because the demonstration of high-level abilities in the animal subjects of their own research could cause problems for the scientists themselves (see Section 3.1). We should deal with complex explanations without arbitrary avoidance of terms associated with them, but should be rigorous in our investigations of the phenomena, defining terms carefully and using all necessary controls.

Feelings and Emotions

5

5.1 Affect, Feelings and Emotions

The scientific study of affect concerns emotions, feelings and moods (Fox, 2008) and there has been a rapid increase in scientific publications about affective neuroscience since 2000 (Sander, 2013). A difficulty in the scientific development of this area has been caused by the tendency of many authors to define or refer to these concepts using human subjective terms that are not descriptive. It may be possible for the empathy of another person to allow some understanding of a subjective statement, but objective descriptions are especially desirable when formulating definitions. When we try to use the concept for another species of animal, a lack of objective definition becomes even more of a problem. Hence, even though it is difficult in this subject area, efforts are made here to define the terms in a universally comprehensible way.

Sander agrees with Fox that affect is not just about emotions, saying that affect includes moods and 'affective dispositions'. Paul *et al.* (2005) state that 'affect involves: behavioural and physiological responses (and in conscious beings, feelings) that can vary both in terms of valence (pleasantness/unpleasantness) and also intensity (arousing/activating qualities)'. If affect were limited to meaning an experiential state involving feelings it could be used only for humans and other animals that can have a sufficient level of awareness to have feelings (Broom, 2010a).

In order to interpret the statements about what affect is, definitions of the constituent phenomena are needed. What exactly are feelings, emotions and moods? Aristotle defined pathê, usually considered to mean emotion or feeling, as 'those things on account of which people change and differ in regard to their judgements, and upon which attend pain and pleasure' (Rhetoric, Book 2, Chapter 1, 1378a). This statement is of particular interest because of the link between judgement and emotion. Other attempts at definition of emotion explain some aspects of the concept but are not comprehensible without examples. For example, James (1894), quoted by Martin and Delgado (2013), said that 'emotions are adaptive behavioural and physiological response tendencies initiated by salient situations or stimuli'. Fox (2008) said that emotions are rather brief and are 'discrete and consistent responses to an internal or external event that has particular significance for the organism'. Rolls (1999) described emotions as states elicited by rewards and punishers while Broom and Fraser (2007) said emotions are 'physiologically describable conditions in individuals characterized by electrical and neuro-chemical activity in particular regions of the brain, autonomic nervous system activity, hormone release and peripheral consequences including behaviour'. However, each of these definitions could include some phenomena that are not emotions. Some stimuli that are rewarding or punishing could lead to several consequences for the individual, spread over a substantial amount of time, some of which – but not others – would be emotions. Sander (2013) does not present a simple definition but agrees with Le Doux (1995) that emotions are conscious states. He summarizes emotions as: (i) being multi-component; (ii) being two-step in that they are elicited and are a response; (iii) having relevant objects; and (iv) having brief duration. Paul et al. (2005) also emphasize that emotions are 'attached in some way to an object' whereas moods are not. Other descriptions of emotions say what they include, such as anger, joy, sadness, fear, disgust and surprise (Sander, 2013). There is debate in the psychological literature about what should be included as emotions, for example whether or not thirst and sexual behaviour should be considered to be emotions, as proposed by Rolls (1999). Dictionary explanations of emotions and feelings often emphasize that they are different from cognitive or volitional states. Such views are now less tenable scientifically because of the known overlap in function between affect and cognition (see below).

The capability of feeling is sometimes specifically linked to touch sensations, but the word is also used in a more general way. Many feelings are associated with an object. While the words 'emotion' and 'feelings' can sometimes be used interchangeably, feelings are thought of as stemming from the brain and to involve sophisticated processing, while emotions can be described more readily in physiological terms. For example, fear is clearly a feeling but there are bodily changes often associated with fear including increased heart rate, increased sweating, facial movements and a greater tendency to flee. The term 'feeling' encompasses the emotion.

The meaning of the term 'feeling', as discussed in Chapter 1, is of key importance in this discussion. A feeling is a brain construct involving at least perceptual awareness which is associated with a life regulating system, is recognizable by the individual when it recurs and may change behaviour or act as a reinforcer in learning (Broom, 1998). In relation to this definition, emotions were considered to be similar but physiologically describable (Broom, 2007b). Rolls (1999) considered feelings to be the subjective consequences of emotions involving consciousness or awareness. If the concepts of emotions and feelings are so closely overlapping, perhaps emotion should refer to feelings, and be defined as a physiologically describable component of a feeling characterized by electrical and neurochemical activity in particular regions of the brain, autonomic nervous system activity, hormone release and peripheral consequences including behaviour.

An affective state is largely equivalent in meaning to a mood (see Section 5.3). The fact that emotions (and usually also feelings) are associated with an object means that they are likely to involve more information processing than moods, and they may promote certain actions (Paul *et al.*, 2005).

It is not possible to discuss feelings or emotions without consideration of positive feelings and consequent good welfare. However, many scientists cannot bring themselves to use words such as happiness, contentment, joy or good welfare in a scientific document. The reason for this is that it is difficult to measure these states scientifically. How should scientists deal with a situation where measurement is difficult? In most aspects of science, they try to find out how to measure the phenomenon, and if they have a little success, they advertise it widely. In relation to the measurement of feelings, the commoner practice is to deny the existence of the phenomenon and to criticize or denigrate those who try to do so. This is not good science. What scientists should do is to obtain information that will allow them to assess at least the presence or absence of the emotion or feeling, and preferably to quantify it. For many feelings this involves assessing the valence. Valence is the extent of pleasantness or unpleasantness. This might be assessed using measures of strength of preference, or using measures of consequence for the individual. The consequences may be behaviours or physiological states associated with the positive and the absence of the negative.

Following the question of whether or not animals can suffer, posed by Bentham (1789), the importance of feelings, in particular in relation to animal welfare, has been emphasized by Duncan (1993), Dawkins (1993), Panksepp (1998) and many others. The biological basis for feelings and the evolution of feelings have been discussed by these authors and by Cabanac (1979) and Broom (1998, 2001b).

There is much public concern about suffering in humans and in other animals. The concept of suffering is directly linked to that of feelings, and Gregory (2004) said that suffering is 'the mental state associated with unpleasant experiences such as pain malaise, distress, injury and emotional numbness'. However, some unpleasant experiences may not lead to feelings so it is better not to define suffering in this way. Also, the word 'suffering' is not used for very brief negative feelings so the definition used here is: suffering is one or more bad feelings continuing for more than a short period (Broom and Fraser, 2007). The ability to feel pain and to suffer in other ways is generally included among the capabilities of sentient animals.

5.2   Physiological Systems of Emotions and Feelings

During emotions there are physiological changes in the body associated with brain activity, and often also with behaviour modification. Heart-rate variability is reduced during negative and increased during positive emotional changes. This is a result of sympathetic nervous system–adrenal–medullary activity. Several different negative emotions are associated with increases in adrenal cortex production of cortisol or corticosterone, depending on the species. Positive experiences may occur at the same time as increases in cardiac vagal tone. Negative experiences may lead to immunosuppression and positive emotions may occur at the same time as increases in oxytocin production.

Many of the changes in the concentrations of hormones that occur in humans also occur in other mammals, birds, fish and, in some instances, invertebrate animals. However, there is variation in the region of the brain that is involved in the control of the hormone release. This fact has led to the view, expressed by some scientists, that only mammals have emotional systems. The major differences in the brain areas involved in emotional responses have arisen because, in tetrapod vertebrates and especially in mammals, the cerebral cortex has taken over some functions previously located in other parts of the brain. The exceptional learning and cognitive abilities of birds (Chapter 4) are largely controlled by the striatum and not by the cerebral cortex as in humans and other mammals. Hence it is clear that a different location of control in the brain does not mean a different degree of sophistication of brain mechanism.

The areas of the brain that have been stated as essential for awareness in mammals are the neural connections between the thalamus and the neocortex. More specifically, the upper brainstem between the diencephalic basal ganglia and midbrain roof or tectum integrates the parallel, distributed information from the cortical representations to produce sequentially ordered outputs resulting in behaviour (Seth and Baars, 2004; Seth *et al.*, 2005). However, as Kirkwood (2006) points out, an argument based on the anatomy of mammals but not on that of birds is unconvincing when some birds have such impressive cognitive ability. In mammals, the control of emotional responses (i.e. the limbic system) is located in the amygdala, the septal nuclei, the hippocampus, and the prefrontal, cingulate and insular cortex (see review by Boissy *et al.*, 2007). Sensory systems have direct links to the limbic system. For example, olfactory nuclei project directly to the amygdala, as does the centre that relays acoustic signals, the medial geniculate body. Positive emotional states, which are generally associated with reward during learning, are associated with the amygdala and the nucleus accumbens septi. Opioids are involved in some of these positive emotional states and, based on studies of feeding, Berridge (1996) suggested that the two different ways in which they affect the dopaminergic systems may indicate that there is a 'wanting system', involving appetite and incentive, and a 'liking system' involving pleasure. Some of the amygdala centres are linked to oxytocin activity. Behaviour that indicates positive and negative emotions is described in Chapter 8.

Fish have a hypothalamic–pituitary–interrenal response that is almost identical to the hypothalamic–pituitary–adrenal (HPA) response of mammals. Stimuli that are disturbing to fish elicit the production of adrenaline and noradrenaline from the chromaffin tissue (Perry and Bernier, 1999). At the same time, corticotrophin-releasing hormone (CRH) is released from the hypothalamus; it leads to release of adrenocorticotrophic hormone (ACTH) from the pituitary; and this, in turn, is carried by the blood to the interrenal tissue, an analogue of the mammalian adrenal gland, where cortisol is produced (Sumpter, 1997; Huntingford *et al.*, 2006).

The brains of fish are very variable in structure. Indeed the mammals can reasonably be considered to have just one of a range of the brain structures that the various evolutionary lines of fish possess. The neocortex is not present in fish so the cortex–thalamic links of mammals cannot exist. This led Rose (2002) to state that absence of such connections means that fish cannot feel pain or have other feelings. However, brains can function in the same ways with the participation of different anatomical areas of the brain. All fish and other vertebrates have a thalamus and connections between this and the striatal area, the optic sensory area on the roof of the midbrain and the telencephalic pallium (Butler and Hodos, 2005). The upper brain stem in humans who lack a cerebral cortex takes on some of its functions so that these people are conscious (Merker, 2007). The anatomical argument for restricting pain and other feelings to mammals is illogical.

The general physiological functioning of cephalopods is impressive: for example, their food conversion efficiency is significantly greater than that of mammals (Boyle, 1987). They have an adrenal system and release adrenal hormones in response to situations that would elicit pain and distress in humans (Broom, 1998, 2001b; Stefano *et al.*, 1998, 2002). They secrete noradrenaline and dopamine in response to disturbing events (e.g. air exposure, food withdrawal).

5.3 Mood

Feelings and emotions are often discussed together with moods and the *Oxford English Dictionary* (2011) defines 'mood' as a frame of mind or state of feelings. Moods include 'frames of mind' that may not be feelings, but what is a frame of mind, and how should the word's meaning be limited? It is more precise to refer to a state of the brain than to use the word 'mind' but it is not clear what level of brain processing is involved when we refer to a mood.

Where there are feelings, some complex analysis must occur, but substantial, low-level brain activity such as a high degree of perceptual processing might be sufficient to define a mood. A further aspect of the meaning is temporal. Factors affecting moods tend to persist, so moods endure over time (Nettle and Bateson, 2012). Rolls (2005) says that a mood state could be produced as a result of the initiation of an emotion but that the mood is not directed towards an object, as the emotion is. However, a mood could also be produced without the emotion, or at least without continuing emotion, and continues for longer than an emotion.

Some moods are referred to using words that imply that a feeling is involved, for example 'anxious', 'fearful', 'happy' or 'contented'. A second category may or may not involve feelings, for example 'tranquil' or 'excited', while a third category such as 'optimistic', 'pessimistic' or 'analytical' would not normally include feelings.

What are the consequences of a mood? Moods can affect activity levels, attention state, sensory functioning, or cognitive processing. Some moods may result in more or less efficient analytical processing and decisions may be affected by mood. For example, a feeling of vulnerability can affect judgement. A definition is: a mood is a brain state that often involves feelings, continues for more than a few minutes and influences decision making and behaviour.

5.4   Cognition in Relation to Emotion

Many studies show how activity in particular regions of the brains of mammals, for example the amygdala, prefrontal and orbitofrontal cortex, anterior cingulate, insula, nucleus accumbens, ventral tegmental area and periaqueductal grey, is associated with emotion and feelings (Panksepp, 1998; Rolls, 2005; Murray, 2007). These authors also report the cognitive components of processes involving emotion. The effects of emotional states on cognition are described in humans and, recently, in some other species (Call and Carpenter, 2001; Paul et al., 2005; Mendl et al., 2009) and may have adaptive value (Mineka et al., 1998; Mendl et al., 2010a). However, in attempts to demonstrate mood-dependent memory, the number of studies that did so was about the same as the number that did not (Eich and Macaulay, 2000). This is not surprising as it would not be adaptive for all learning and memory to be mood-dependent. Rolls (1999) argues that cognitive and emotional mechanisms are closely linked because reward systems are important in the control of life, and reward is often associated with emotional responses. He uses the term 'emotional behaviour' for the goal-directed actions when working for rewards. In some cases, working to avoid aversive stimuli or negative reinforcement also involves emotions, for example the feeling of fear in humans (Scherer, 1999) and fear and other feelings in farm animals (Dantzer, 2002). Negative feelings associated with decreased sensitivity to reward, referred to as 'anhedonia-like', are described to show reduced anticipation of rewarding stimuli, such as sweet foods (Spruijt et al., 2001).

The key question of whether emotional and cognitive systems are distinct is discussed by Paul *et al.* (2005). It has been thought by some that cognition is nothing to do with emotion, but this view is contradicted by many studies reported here. Panksepp (2003) argued that cognitive processes are inextricably linked to emotional processes, but regarded them as essentially distinct and independent in function. Referring to mammals, Panksepp considered cognitive mechanisms as cortical in location but affective systems as largely sub-cortical. A quite different view is that of Forgas (2000) who argued that an emotional response must be preceded by identification of a stimulus and that emotional responses involve cognitive components. Clore and Ortony (2000) state that changes in informational processes with cognitive components are integral parts of emotional processes. The validity of this point depends on the definition of cognition. With the very broad definition of Shettleworth (2010), there must be a cognition component in the perception involved in emotional responses. Even with the narrower definition of cognition used here, it is difficult to envisage feelings occurring without the complex analytical learning and evaluation processes that would involve cognition. If, as described above, cognition involves having a concept of something in its absence, since feelings are not switched off suddenly at the end of a perception, they would also seem very likely to involve cognition. Emotion might sometimes be simpler than a feeling but the fact that it is describable in terms of physiology and subsequent behaviour would not prevent it from having a cognitive component.

The phenomenon of cognitive bias is discussed in Section 4.9, rather than in this chapter, because the phenomenon itself is to do with information processing, decision making and cognition. Its occurrence is altered by affect, but also by components of mood and other factors that are not to do with feelings. A further link between emotion and cognition is the effect of emotional state on what is learned. Carey and Fry (1993, 1995) trained pigs to show an operant response when in a drug-induced anxious state and a different operant response when in a normal state. The pigs indicated drug presence by their response. They also made this 'drug-present' response when anxiety was induced by exposure to a novel pen, a novel object, transportation or exposure to an unfamiliar pig that might be threatening. The learning studies, with their associated cognitive change, gave results that provided information about the emotional state of the pigs.

Rolls (1999) explains how the orbital–frontal cortex in the primate brain is used to compute the value of resources and actions. In other mammals, such as rodents, there is no orbital–frontal cortex, so Rolls asks whether or not they have the capacity to compute value. Another example of differences between these two animal groups is that taste pathways go to the cortex in humans but to the hypothalamus and amygdala in rodents. We need more information about the brain mechanisms underlying affect and value determination in the different kinds of brains that are found among animal species.

5.5 Pain

The pain system includes both simple sensory aspects and complex brain analysis. Pain receptors are often called nociceptors, and it is useful to have a specific term for them that distinguishes their input to the pain pathways from that of other kinds of receptor. In humans, nociception is considered by some to be the physiological relay of pain signals: an involuntary, reflex process not involving awareness. It would seem that the distinction between nociception and pain is a relic of attempts to emphasize differences between humans and other animals or between 'higher' and 'lower' animals. The visual and auditory systems involve receptors, pathways and high-level analysis in the brain, but the simpler and more complex aspects are not given different names. A perception of pain can exist without the involvement of pain receptors, but visual or auditory perceptions can also exist without their receptors being involved. Wall (1992) said that the problem of pain in man and animals was 'confused by the pseudoscience surrounding the word nociception'. The use of the term 'nociception', which separates one part of the pain system from other parts, should be discontinued; the system should be considered as a whole (Broom, 2001a).

Pain leads to aversion; that is, to behavioural responses involving immediate avoidance and learning to avoid a similar situation or stimulus later. Pain has a sensory component often related to injury but also requires complex brain functioning of the kind associated with a feeling. Based on the International Association for the Study of Pain definition (Iggo, 1984), Kavaliers (1989) suggested that for non-humans, pain is 'an aversive sensory experience caused by actual or potential injury that elicits protective motor and vegetative reactions, results in learned avoidance and may modify species specific behaviour, including social behaviour'. More simply, Smith and Boyd (1991) considered pain to be the conscious, emotional experience that, in humans, involves nerve pathways in the cerebrum. Hence a definition of pain should refer to the sensory and emotional aspects, and the reference to function and consequences is not needed as it may unnecessarily restrict its meaning. Accordingly, Broom's (2001b) definition was: pain is an aversive sensation and feeling associated with actual or potential tissue damage.

If pain occurs in an animal, it can cause poor welfare. Among animals that can feel pain, the degree of awareness will vary. However, understanding pain is important for each kind of animal because many people consider that the protection of a group of animals is not necessary unless one of their capabilities is to be able to feel pain.

Many kinds of aquatic and terrestrial animals have a pain system involving receptors, neural pathways and analytical centres in the brain. There is also evidence from many animal groups of physiological responses, direct behavioural responses and ability to learn from such experiences so that they are minimized or avoided in future. This suggests the existence of feelings of pain in many species. Feelings such as pain, fear and various kinds of pleasure will often be an important part of the biological mechanism for coping with actual or potential damage. Sometimes the response is to avoid whatever is causing the damage. Consequent learning allows the minimizing of future damage and, where the pain is chronic, behaviour and physiology can be changed to ameliorate adverse effects. Pain systems have been identified by anatomical and physiological investigation and by studies of behavioural responses, particularly with the assistance of analgesic administration as an experimental probe.

Species differ in their responses to painful stimuli: for example, dogs and humans make much noise but sheep do not, because loud vocalizations may elicit help from social group members in dogs and humans but just attract more predator attention to an injured sheep. Hence different responses are adaptive in different species. The feeling of pain may be the same even if the responses are very different. Immediate responses may vary but avoidance of the painful stimulus, and the effects on subsequent responses of learning to avoid such stimuli, should be observable in any animal that feels pain. Careful observation and experiment have also allowed other feelings such as fear, anxiety and the various forms of pleasure to be deduced to exist.

How should we decide whether or not an animal can feel pain? Patrick Bateson (1991) proposed that an animal showing behaviour and physiology homologous with humans undergoing pain and suffering should be treated as suffering unless there is evidence to the contrary. This approach is similar to the use of the precautionary principle for wider areas of animal ability proposed by Harry Bradshaw (Bradshaw, 1998) and others.

The occurrence of pain in fish is debated by Broom (2001b), Rose (2002), Jackson (2003), Chandroo *et al.* (2004) and Braithwaite and Huntingford (2004). In the rainbow trout *Onchorhynchus mykiss*, anatomical and electrophysiological investigation of the nociceptors connected to the trigeminal nerve has revealed that these fish have two types of nociceptor, A-delta and c fibres (Sneddon, 2002; Sneddon *et al.*, 2003a). The transmitter substance P is typical of pain systems in mammals and in fish. The encephalins and β-endorphin, which are opioids and act as endogenous analgesics in mammals, are present in fish (Rodriguez-Moldes *et al.*, 1993; Zaccone *et al.*, 1994; Balm and Pottinger, 1995) and the behavioural responses of goldfish to analgesics are the same as in rats (Ehrensing *et al.*, 1982). When Sneddon *et al.* (2003b) administered weak acetic acid solution or bee venom to the mouth of a trout, the fish rested on the substratum, rocked from side to side and rubbed their snouts on solid surfaces. These behaviours stopped when the analgesic morphine was given. It is clear that fish have a pain system whose function is very similar to that of mammals. There are, as mentioned above, differences in the location in the brain of the area where the information is analysed.

Cephalopods have nociceptors that respond maximally to an injurious stimulus, but not to an innocuous stimulus, and increase their sensitivity after tissue has been injured to help the animal avoid further injury. There is also some indication that their rate of firing or sensitivity is related to the sensitivity of the tissue which they protect (Mather, 2004). They can learn to avoid putatively painful stimuli (Young, 1991) and have many of the neurotransmitters that are involved in vertebrate pain reception and mediation (Abbott *et al.*, 1995).

Octopuses have been trained to withdraw from or alter their behaviour in response to a conditioned stimulus when this has been previously paired with an electric shock (Robertson *et al.*, 1995). If a vertebrate species is used in such studies, it is usually taken for granted that the learning process has arisen as the result of the animal experiencing pain or discomfort from the electric shock.

Many other invertebrate animals have elements of a pain system (Sherwin, 2001; Broom, 2013). Decapod crustaceans show behavioural, anatomical and physiological indications of having a sophisticated pain system. They have nociceptors that supply information to ganglia involved in learning (Sandeman *et al.*, 1992). Avoidance learning to noxious stimuli occurs in crayfish (Kawai *et al.*, 2004) and sand lobsters (Sherwin, 2001). Analgesic opioids affecting responses and learning have been reported in animals such as shrimps and crabs by Maldonado and Miralto (1982), Lozda *et al.* (1988) and Bergamo *et al.* (1992). Naloxone inhibits the opioid action, as in vertebrates (Dyakonova, 2001).

Elwood and colleagues (Barr *et al.*, 2008; Elwood *et al.*, 2009; Elwood and Appel, 2009; Elwood, 2012, 2013) found that prawns whose antennae were treated with acid or alkali showed increased antennal cleaning movements, but these were not shown if an anaesthetic had been used prior to treatment. They also described how crabs normally preferred to stay in shelter but learned after two trials to avoid a shelter where they had received shocks. Hermit crabs in non-preferred *Gibbula* (top-shell) shells were more likely to leave the shell when shocked than if they were in a preferred *Littorina* (winkle) shell. Since they were trading off the preference and the negative experience, the authors concluded that pain rather than nociception was indicated.

Leeches such as *Hirudo* have mechanoreceptors that fulfil the criteria for nociceptors. It is likely that many other invertebrates have such receptors. However, vertebrate animals utilize both specialist nociceptors and normal receptors to gain information about actual or potential tissue damage. Hence, while the presence of specialist nociceptors is evidence for the presence of part of a pain system, their absence does not mean that no pain sensation can occur. Behavioural avoidance of sources of potential or actual tissue damage is shown by sea anemones, earthworms and most other invertebrate animals (Smith and Boyd, 1991). However, this does not tell us that they feel the consequences of damage. It is of interest that leeches and the swimming sea slug *Aplysia* are used as models in vertebrate pain studies (Woolf and Walters, 1991). Clearly the similarities in the components of the pain system that they possess are sufficient for extrapolation to vertebrates. Studies of humans, mice and the fruit fly *Drosophila* have revealed the existence of genes that seem to be involved in aspects of pain in each animal (Neely *et al.*, 2011).

The receptors, transmission system and some analysis that could be part of a pain system are reported from many invertebrate groups, for example earthworms and other annelids, gastropod molluscs and insects

(Stefano *et al.*, 2002). Insects poisoned with DDT, or restrained, often struggle or show convulsions. Such a reaction could indicate pain but may not. If an animal has a substantial injury but continues to show attempts to carry out normal movements, does this mean that it does not feel pain consequent upon the injury? Several insect species have been observed to continue walking after their foot has been crushed. Locusts may continue eating when being consumed by a praying mantis, and aphids may do the same when eaten by a coccinelid (ladybird) beetle (Eisner, 1993). This may mean that they feel no pain but there are parallels with mammals that do not show active responses when predators injure them, even when physiological responses characteristic of pain are occurring (Broom, 2001a). The avoidance of an active response can be adaptive and save the life of the individual. Spiders such as *Argiope* (Fiorito, 1986) can respond to mechanical pressure on the body by autotomizing limbs. So can some insects, while lizards may autotomize the tail. This does not tell us that these animals do or do not feel pain.

Although opioids have an important role in the natural regulation of mammalian pain, they have many different functions in animals, almost certainly with some differences in the various phyla. Earthworms show wriggling and escape responses when injured, and these responses are suppressed by naloxone, an opioid inhibitor. Honeybees (*Apis mellifera*) and praying mantis (*Stagmatophora biocellata*) are among the insects known to produce opioids during defensive reactions and to have opioid receptors that are blocked by naloxone, as in humans and other vertebrates. Snails (*Cepaea nemoralis*) lift part of their foot if it is in contact with a surface that is being warmed to 40°C (Kavaliers and Hirst, 1983). Several opioids have been found to inhibit this response. Slugs and other molluscs have opioids and naloxone inhibits their action. It is unlikely that the opioid systems have arisen independently during the evolution of the various invertebrates and the vertebrates. Hence it is probable that opioids are playing a role in the pain response of many invertebrate animals.

Ross and Ross (2009) have produced a book that includes a variety of methods for using anaesthesia and analgesia for invertebrate animals. Some anaesthetics suppress movement in a way that would be useful for a veterinary surgeon or experimenter. However, such a book would be of little use if there were no pain in these animals. Analgesic action does imply that pain is occurring but in many cases we do not know how analgesics or anaesthetic are acting. As with humans and other vertebrates, stopping responses to tissue damage does not necessarily mean that there is pain or that pain is stopped. A worm or mollusc that is injured, and perhaps writhing, may be feeling pain but could be showing an automatic response. The change in scientific thinking is that the weight of evidence for some of these animals now indicates that they may be feeling pain. Walters and Moroz (2009) review evidence for memory of injury in molluscs, principally *Aplysia*. If these animals can remember injury, their experience must be close to pain.

5.6   Fear

Fear is a feeling that occurs when there is perceived to be actual danger or a risk of danger. Fear involves more complex analysis than just a startle response, in that current sensory input is compared with previously experienced events (Broom, 1998). Behavioural and emotional fear responses in mammals involve the amygdala, the peri-aqueductal grey of the midbrain and the hypothalamus. The responses when fear is felt may be to remain immobile or to make vigorous attempts to escape, depending upon the species feeling the fear, the stimuli eliciting it and the previous experience of that individual in such circumstances. Fear is often reported by humans to be associated with very poor welfare and more extreme in its consequences than most pain.

5.7   Anxiety

The identification of anxiety in humans usually depends on: (i) what people report about their feelings in particular circumstances; (ii) what clinical effects can be observed; and (iii) the consequences of the use of drugs described as being anxiolytic on (i) and (ii). However, some anxieties are not often reported; some people are loath to report any anxiety at all; and some anxieties may occur without detectable clinical effects. Hence anxiety may often be missed. A further problem is that people may report a low level of anxiety as being a high level and may even simulate anxiety effects in order to achieve a social objective.

The testing of anxiolytic drugs is carried out on laboratory animals, so it is assumed that anxiety occurs in these animals in much the same way as it does in humans. Many of these drugs are used in veterinary medicine as well as in human medicine. Studies of the behaviour of domestic and laboratory animals in situations where there are uncertainties that are important to the individuals tested also indicate that anxiety is a widespread feeling among non-human animals.

5.8   Various Pleasures

Cabanac (1979) suggested that many behavioural or physiological responses that involve a return to homeostasis are associated with pleasure: for example if an animal has become cold and is able to be in a warm place, as in the case of Japanese macaques bathing in a natural hot pool in cold weather. Similarly, food and water after deprivation may lead to pleasure and it may be either high or low arousal. In most of the studies that suggest this, the responses measured that indicate the existence of pleasure are largely behavioural, but some physiological responses have also been measured (Broom, 2010a). Behavioural studies indicating that individuals feel pleasure include that of Widowski and

Duncan (2000), who argue that dust-bathing in hens is motivated by pleasure. Physiological changes associated with pleasure include certain vagal nerve activations and increases in oxytocin concentrations. Oxytocin is involved in nursing behaviour in lactating female mammals. Human mothers describe nursing as pleasurable and oxytocin is elevated at this time. However, oxytocin concentration is also elevated in several other circumstances that seem likely to involve pleasure (Carter, 2001) (see Chapter 8).

Exploration or seeking is listed as a positive feeling by some authors (Panksepp, 2005; Mellor, 2011). Much of exploration will involve controlled movements around an area and expectation of specific inputs relevant to the capacity of the individual to control its interactions with its environment. This activity may involve positive feelings but need not do so. Exploration could occur in dangerous situations where the net impact on the individual is negative. In other circumstances, the expectations of obtaining a positive experience may be high, so the net feeling is positive.

5.9   Social Affection

Affiliative behaviour between parents and offspring, or between other individuals, has the effect of promoting bonding and is associated with positive feelings. Oxytocin and vasopressin can promote affiliative behaviour (Nelson and Panksepp, 1998). The brain regions involved in social affection in mammals include the anterior cingulate cortex, the bed nucleus of the stria terminalis, the dorsomedial thalamus, the ventral septal and preoptic areas, and the periaqueductal grey of the brainstem.

5.10   Guilt, Anger and Rage

Guilt is a feeling that is associated with a perception of having done wrong. Carla Torres-Pereira observed pet dogs that had been told by their owners not to take a food object (Fig. 5.1). When the owner then left the room (Fig. 5.2), some dogs ate the food object. These dogs had a higher heart rate than dogs that obeyed. When the owner returned after 30 s and carefully avoided looking at the dog, there was a difference in behaviour between dogs that had taken the food and those that had not. The existence of the concept of wrongness, which cannot be separated from an association of an action with predicted negative consequences, is implied by these results (Torres-Pereira and Broom, 2010).

Anger or rage is a feeling that is generally considered negative, in particular because of its consequences. The areas of the brain that are active during this feeling are the medial hypothalamus and the peri-aqueductal grey, and there are often inputs from the amygdala. This anatomical distribution is very similar to that during fear and the two feelings overlap in the circumstances of elicitation. The neural control and elicitation mechanism are different.

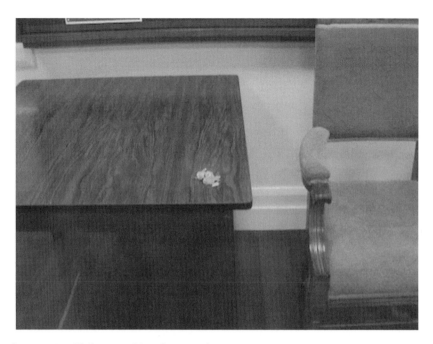

Fig. 5.1. Food left on a table (photograph C.M.C. Torres-Pereira).

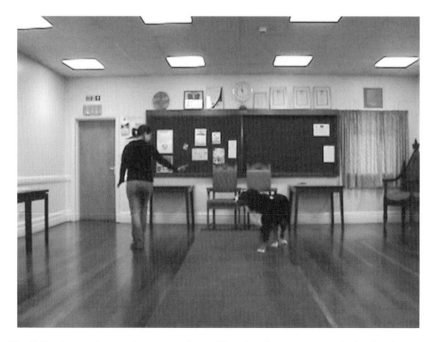

Fig. 5.2. Owner leaves the room after telling the dog not to touch the food (photograph C.M.C. Torres-Pereira).

5.11 Welfare in Relation to Feelings

Pain, fear and other negative feelings that contribute to suffering have long been seen as important subjects to investigate in animal welfare research and, more recently, the occurrence of positive feelings has been an aim (Broom and Johnson, 1993; Carter, 2001; Boissy *et al.*, 2007). However, researchers have often hesitated to say that they were trying to assess feelings. Experimental studies that indicate the occurrence of feelings have been described more and more often in recent years. Studies directed towards quantifying the occurrence of pain and malaise in animals and descriptions of methods for their alleviation have been presented by many authors (e.g. Stafford *et al.*, 2003; Gregory, 2004; Stilwell *et al.*, 2008). References to other feelings in welfare research have been cautious. For example, Désiré *et al.* (2002, 2004, 2006) studied sheep disturbed by the sudden appearance of a coloured scarf. They recorded several behavioural responses, heart-rate changes and modification of vagal tone measured by the rate of firing in the vagal nerve. The behavioural and physiological responses occurred if the timing and nature of the appearance of the scarf were predictable. However, they increased when the presentation was sudden rather than gradual, and increased in proportion to how unfamiliar and how large the stimulus was. These are the factors that would affect the likelihood of fear in humans so the authors concluded that sheep feel fear in such situations.

Awareness and Consciousness

6

6.1 The Meaning of Awareness

Some psychologists and neuroscientists assume that among all vertebrates and invertebrates, only mammals have the abilities that make up sentience. For example, Panksepp (1998), in a figure on page 35 of his valuable book *Affective Neuroscience*, assumes that awareness is limited to mammals and reflexive behaviour starts with reptiles, while fish are depicted as having no ability. He describes some of the relatively complex behaviour of the swimming sea slug *Aplysia*, including responses to punishment, but assumes that all is 'preconscious' and automatic. Even birds have often been excluded from discussions of awareness or consciousness.

The desirability of scientific investigation of awareness in non-human animals was emphasized by Griffin (1984). The concept of awareness has been discussed extensively in relation to humans and other species (Burghardt, 1985) but few have attempted to define it. There may be confusion between consciousness and awareness (see Section 6.2, below). As mentioned in Chapter 1, Broom (1998) defined awareness as a state in which complex brain analysis is used to process sensory stimuli or constructs based on memory. This definition limits the characteristics of the state but does not describe what the phenomenon is. Hence it is necessary to explain that key parts of awareness are the concepts that the individual has about its environment, itself, and itself in relation to relevant aspects of its environment. Some of the various aspects of such concepts are discussed further in this chapter. The definition of aware-ness is changed here to: a state during which concepts of environment, of self, and of self in relation to environment result from complex brain analysis of sensory stimuli or constructs based on memory.

One of the difficulties when referring to awareness is that there is a range of complexities of brain processing encompassed within the concept. An indi-vidual may be aware of a simple change in its environment, such as the increase in light level at dawn, but may also be aware of another individual having, or not having, a particular concept. Different kinds of animal and different indi-viduals may have the capacity to be aware in a simple way but not in a more complex way. As a consequence, several kinds, levels or degrees of awareness have been described. In categorizing awareness a hierarchy has usually been suggested. It may also be assumed that the different kinds of awareness have arisen at different times during animal evolution. However, there can be dif-ferences in awareness that are qualitative but with no certainty about degree of complexity of functioning involved. While more complex processing would normally occur chronologically later in evolution than simpler processing, dif-ferent kinds of processing could arise independently, and could arise in differ-ent parts of the brain and more than once. Awareness could be categorized in many ways. Hence the word used below for different kinds of awareness is 'categories' rather than 'levels'.

Human experience, such as touch, smell, joy or sorrow, are aspects of awareness that seem to be independent of language, and hence such aware-ness might be common to linguistic and non-linguistic animals (Damasio, 2000; Mendl and Paul, 2004).

There have been many attempts to categorize awareness or conscious-ness. One of the most influential is the Buddhist division of concepts, on the one hand, into present and future; and on the other hand, into self and the outside world (Crook, 1988). These areas of awareness are discussed fur-ther in Sections 6.4–6.7. In an attempt to consider how different awareness might involve different complexities of brain processing, awareness has been described using five categories: unaware, perceptual awareness, cognitive awareness, assessment awareness and executive awareness (Sommerville and Broom, 1998). In perceptual awareness, a stimulus elicits activity in brain centres but the individual may or may not be capable of modifying the response voluntarily (e.g. scratching to relieve irritation). Examples of cognitive aware-ness include a mother recognizing her offspring and an individual responding to a known competitor, ally, dwelling place or food type. An individual is show-ing assessment awareness if it is able to assess and deduce the significance of a situation in relation to itself over a short time span: for example, vertebrate prey responding to a predator recognized as posing an immediate threat but not directly attacking. Executive awareness exists when the individual is able to assess, deduce and plan in relation to long-term intention. In order to have intentions, the individual must have some capability to plan for the future. This requires that information received now can be related to a concept of events that will occur in the future. Executive awareness may involve deductions about choices of action available to that individual (retroduction), the feelings of others, imagination and the mental construction of elaborate sequences of events.

Other attempts to categorize awareness have used other words, in particular 'consciousness' (see Section 6.3). Lunzer (1979) used level 1 to mean awake, level 2 to mean able to form concepts and generalize and level 3 for when an object can be attended to, voluntarily represented and verbally communicated. Level 3 is defined for humans and equates to the access consciousness of Block (1998). Snyder *et al.* (2004) refer to awareness of concepts and equate consciousness with executive awareness. Mendl and Paul (2004, 2008) discuss basic awareness of sensations, feelings, emotions and memories.

A category of 'phenomenal consciousness' has been used (e.g. Allen and Bekoff, 2007) to refer to what is experienced during feelings. Some authors consider that all that is needed for awareness of feelings is for there to be access by other parts of the brain to primary sensory information (Tye, 2000), while others have said that awareness of self is needed before there can be awareness of feelings, or phenomenal consciousness (Carruthers, 2000).

The complexity of brain organization is greater for animals that must contend with a varied environment. Such animals have an elaborate motivational system that allows them to think about the impacts of that environment and then take appropriate decisions. Some kinds of feeding methods and predator avoidance demand a great cognitive capacity, but the most demanding thing in life for humans and many other species is to live and organize behaviour effectively in a social group (Broom, 1981a, 2003; Humphrey, 1986, 1992). Animals that live socially are generally more complex in their functioning and in their cognitive capacity than related animals that are not social. When deciding whether animals are sentient, a first step is the analysis of the degree of complexity of living that is possible for the members of the species (Broom, 2007a). Without a level of brain functioning that makes some degree of awareness possible (Sommerville and Broom, 1998), an animal could not normally be sentient.

6.2   Reporting Perception and Blind-sight

What people report that they perceive is not always what they actually perceive. This can occur because the person is attempting to deceive the listener. In the same way, non-human animals may act as if they see or hear danger when there is none, in order to obtain a resource or social advantage. Reporting is often entirely honest but may sometimes be honest but misled. People with brain injuries who are conscious, in the sense of being awake, may be aware of some environmental events but not others that would normally be perceived by a person. Weiskrantz (1997) reported that such human patients with damage to an area of the striate cortex in the brain say that they are blind in a part of the visual field connected to that area. However, such persons who report that they see nothing may be able to answer questions that indicate that they have obtained information about the stimuli that they deny seeing. Weiskrantz (1997) also described this phenomenon in brain-damaged monkeys and called it blind-sight.

There are also studies of other amnesia patients who state, and clearly believe, that they have forgotten about events but can be demonstrated to have some memory of them. An important result of studies of blind-sight and related phenomena is that, presumably because of alternative neural pathways, monkeys and people with damage that completely prevents output from that brain area can respond to visual stimuli in the corresponding area of the visual field. A person with such damage could show good visual discrimination but be unable to report anything about the experience. Weiskrantz also reports that a human patient with no sensation of touch in the right side of the body, caused by lesions in the left parietal lobe of the brain, when blindfolded and touched on the right side could point to the locus of stimulation. In each of these cases there is a loss of aspects of awareness, but it is clear that sensory functioning is still occurring. Some authors have suggested that there is a general awareness module in the brain, but as Weiskrantz points out there is no evidence from patients with brain damage for the existence of such a module. Indeed, the absence of awareness of some type of sensory input does not mean that there is any deficiency in other aspects of awareness. Also, it seems possible that, where there is damage to an area of the striate cortex, the high-level brain processing associated with awareness of sensory events in the relevant visual area is still occurring in some part of the brain but is blocked by an output associated with the damage (Broom, 2003). However, as Mendl *et al.* (2004) point out, the parallels between humans and monkeys in the occurrence of blind-sight are informative and the studies suggest that there are two levels of cognitive processing.

6.3 Consciousness

People talk about consciousness in different ways. During an operation in a hospital, or after being involved in an accident, a decision about whether or not an individual is conscious is usually determined by the presence or absence of responses to stimuli. It is then normally assumed that the full range of capacity for awareness and cognition is available to the individual. With this logic, a non-anaesthetized human has the full range of human abilities so is conscious, both in the sense of being capable of receiving sensory information and with the meaning of having executive awareness. A normal person, a senile person, a mouse and a trout would all be called conscious on recovery from anaesthesia. However, if the discussion were different and concerned the capacity of the individual to feel pain or pleasure, or to have the most sophisticated awareness, scientists might not classify all four of these as conscious.

It is clear from this that the term 'conscious' has at least two meanings, the second being largely equivalent to 'aware'. As Burghardt (2009) points out, many people who use the word 'conscious' mean one thing on one occasion and another thing on another occasion. It is confusing to have multiple meanings for a term, and especially confusing to use them during one argument, or even during one sentence.

The range of ways in which people have used 'consciousness' is discussed by Broom (2003) and Seth *et al.* (2005). An example of the widespread medical and veterinary use, mentioned above and in Section 1.4, is that of Blood and Studdert (1988) who define conscious as: 'capable of responding to sensory stimuli; awake; aware'. At the other extreme Damasio *et al.* (2000) say that consciousness of an emotion corresponds to knowledge of the ability to experience emotions. This subtle ability refers to perceptual, or anoetic, consciousness: the capacity to be aware of feelings, sensations, thoughts and emotions (Block, 1991). A result of the confusing way in which people have written about consciousness is that it has sometimes been defined by reference to another term. O'Flanagan (1992) defines 'consciousness' as mental states or events that involve awareness. If that were the meaning, since awareness involves mental states, the word 'consciousness' would seem redundant. Another use of the word for only sophisticated ability is that of Gallup (1983) who refers to consciousness as 'the demonstrable capacity to reflect about the self, specifically the ability to recognize oneself in mirrors'. Most people, however, would not think about whether individuals can recognize themselves in a mirror when deciding whether or not they are conscious. As Weiskrantz (1997) puts it: 'no one would have a problem in declaring that a comatose animal is unconscious'.

I consider that it would be better to limit the word 'conscious' to one meaning and that this should be that the individual is not anaesthetized or otherwise caused to be unconscious. The other meanings of 'conscious' could then be expressed by reference to 'awareness', as this term is more readily understood to involve different categories or levels. A conscious individual is one that has the capability to perceive and respond to sensory stimuli. The word 'perceive' implies substantial brain analysis of input and does not just mean 'detect'. This definition is close in concept to the statement by Dawkins (2006): '"Consciousness" usually refers to a wide range of states in which there is an immediate awareness of thought, image or sensation.' The word 'immediate' suggests that Dawkins intended to emphasize the difference from unconscious. Another point that is raised is the distinction between a conscious individual and an individual that is dreaming and might be to some extent aware of thoughts or images. The reference to capability of responding in my definition excludes dreaming.

If the meaning of 'consciousness' is limited as suggested above, the problems described by Marian Dawkins (2012), who considers that there should not be emphasis on whether or not animals have conscious experiences when their welfare is discussed, are solved for the word 'conscious'. However, they are passed instead to what is meant by awareness. While I argue that welfare can be assessed whether or not the individual is aware, there is no doubt that many people would only wish to legally protect animals that are sentient, and hence aware. They might also have more concern about humans who are aware (see Chapter 9). As there is also enormous interest in awareness and sentience, it is not possible to divorce concerns about how animals should be treated from these issues.

6.4   Assessing Own Actions and the Actions of Others

To what extent can individuals use information resulting from their own actions? All animals have some kinds of sensory ability and some analytical capacity to change responses according to what is detected after an action. The control of movement depends on such ability, as do simple food-finding and harm-avoidance mechanisms. As explained in Chapter 4, learning and memory in almost all animals allow flexible responses to the environment and to own actions within that environment. The issue here is the extent to which there is awareness of own actions and of self in relation to the environment that may or may not be changed by them.

When observing another individual, it is useful to have the ability to evaluate the effects of that individual on the environment that it shares with the observer: for example, consuming food or creating danger. In order to do this, the observer has to have a concept of the other individual as something that can act independently of the observer and can have effects on its environment. There must also be not only direct awareness of the relevant parts of the environment, but potentially also a concept of them when they are not (directly at least) observable. If another individual appears to be taking food that is out of sight, the observer needs to know this and evaluate the significance of what is observed. In a social environment, the actions of others may alter social relationships, so assessment of these may be crucially important to the observer. For example, the individual observed may be approaching, or signalling to, a third individual that is a potential mate for both observer and observed.

The evidence that socially living fish can assess the actions of others is clear (Huntingford *et al.*, 2006). Memory in fish is described in many papers and books (Laming, 1981; Huntingford *et al.*, 2006). Fish often live in hazardous environments and have to be able to evaluate the risks associated with carrying out certain activities, going to certain places and consuming certain foods (Yue *et al.*, 2004). Awareness in fish is discussed by Chandroo *et al.* (2004) and Broom (2007a).

The conditioning that has been shown in marine sea slugs (Section 4.6) would require at least cognitive awareness. Place learning by cockroaches and the formation of cognitive maps by bees and ants involve at least assessment awareness. Predatory fireflies *Photuris* mimic the signals of other firefly species, attract males and eat them. The flashing pattern used in this deception is changed to that of another potential prey species if the flashing of that second species is the most frequent in a given location. In addition, when prey use countermeasures, the predator also changes signals and behaviour (Lloyd, 1986). The complexity of these responses cannot be accounted for by automatic processes so quite sophisticated cognitive ability is indicated. Stomatopod crustaceans, such as *Squilla*, also use deception in contests with other individuals (Caldwell, 1986).

In studies of the jumping spider *Portia*, Jackson and Wilcox (1994) and Wilcox and Jackson (1998) have found them to have a very sophisticated ability to evaluate when to jump, to assess where to jump accurately onto the prey and also to show deception and modify movements in accordance with the circumstances. During predation on other spiders, *Portia* and other arachnophagic species deceive the prey while gaining information that optimizes their attack strategy (Jackson and Wilcox, 1992; Jackson and Cross, 2011). When a *Portia* individual is preparing to attack another spider, it is clear that a sequence of movements is planned and then detours are executed which increase the chances of success (Cross and Jackson, 2005). These spiders must have some awareness of themselves in relation to the environment and of an event that is expected in the future such as the jump onto the prey (Jackson and Cross, 2011), so executive awareness is once again implied. Rolls (2005) argues that the ability to exhibit flexible planning is evidence that the individual is not just using automatic brain systems but is conscious or aware of the world around it. If this is the threshold criterion for complexity of cognitive function then these spiders are aware. The cognitive ability they exhibit is great but they require a much longer time for the brain analysis than would a vertebrate, which has a much larger brain. The occurrence of play behaviour, suggested as evidence for assessment awareness, is described for a spider species in Section 8.4.

6.5   Concepts of the Future

As explained by Broom and Fraser (2007), body-state control may occur by negative feedback or by feedforward control, in which a displacement from the tolerable range is predicted and a correction is made before the state changes. Research on animal behaviour is providing more and more evidence of feedforward control in operation. For example, a person expecting to get colder when leaving a warm place will put on more clothes; a cow expecting a period without food will eat more food before this happens; and an individual pig or human entering a room in which there are potentially aggressive individuals will move in such a way that the likelihood of any attack is minimized. The realization that animals often predict likely changes in body temperature, body nutrient levels or social actions has resulted in our view of animals changing to one of them as cognitive beings aware of the complexities of their environment.

Many responses to perceived environmental changes are not just related to that change but also involve predictions about what will happen next. Studies

of animals in learning situations show that they not only associate succes-
sive events, but also assess the probability that events will occur (Dickinson
and Balleine, 2002). As Forkman (2002) says, 'Any animal that can predict
the future has a tremendous advantage over one that cannot. Predicting and
to some extent controlling the future, is really what learning is all about.' If
rats are in a maze and have had previous experience of receiving a particular
reward when they successfully navigate to the end, if that reward is not present
or is inadequate when they get to the end, they show very different behaviour
from that of a rat that reaches the end after no such training. This is evidence
of their expectation of the food reward. They must have a concept of what
reward they are likely to obtain before they get to the normal reward site.

There is also evidence of predictions of the future during the normal life of
animals on farms. Pigs fed at a particular time of day change their behaviour
in the hour before feeding, and cattle show responses if their feed gate does not
work. Previous unpleasant experiences also result in expectation, so a cow that
has experienced unpleasant veterinary treatment in a crush may be unwilling
to enter it later (Broom, 1987); and a sheep that has been roughly or painfully
treated at the end of a race will be difficult to drive into and along that race on
subsequent occasions (Rushen, 1986). Previous experience with stockpersons
can substantially alter later farm animal behaviour and ease of management
by people (Hemsworth and Coleman, 1998).

Expectations about the future are associated with measurable physiological and behavioural changes in humans and other animals. As explained
in Chapter 8, the heart rate of an animal is a useful welfare indicator. When a
problem is predicted, heart rate is increased before the point of requiring the
extra energy availability that increased heart rate brings. Similarly, increased
adrenal activity and hence energetic resources occur when the necessity for
the energy in the near future is perceived, not just when the energy drain
has occurred. Body temperature increases when the adrenal responses have
occurred so a chicken fearing a problem has a higher comb temperature than
a calm chicken. The reverse effect has also been found. A chicken anticipating
that it will receive a palatable reward has a drop in comb temperature at this
time (Moe *et al.*, 2012). The immediate future is a matter of much concern for
sentient animals so they have mechanisms to prepare for it.

As Mendl and Paul (2008) explain, humans frequently engage in 'mental
time travel'. We have episodic memory, which records when things happen as
well as what happens, and also have concepts about what will happen at future
points in time. The description of feedforward control above makes it clear that
non-human animals depend for their functioning on some concepts of future
events. A range of studies, including the work on jumping spiders described in
Section 6.4 above, imply that individuals have an awareness of an action in the
future. Work on animal cognition utilizes methodology that, in primates and
corvids, has demonstrated: (i) prospective thinking, in which several conceptual areas are visited without duplication; (ii) semantic future thinking, where
the individual is shown to envisage the future without the self being involved

in it; and (iii) episodic future thinking, involving personal projection in which the self is part of the future scenario (Raby and Clayton, 2009).

An example of a study showing a concept of time past and future is that of Clayton and Dickinson (1998) who showed that scrub jays that cache food would return earlier to cached waxworms than to cached peanuts, which would not decay as rapidly. Emery and Clayton (2001) also showed that, in a situation where another bird was watching the caching behaviour, scrub jays were more likely to re-cache the food than if they were not observed. The birds that did this must have had a concept that, in the future, the other bird might steal the cached food. When jays had information about which of two foods would be available to them to eat the following day, and were then given the opportunity to cache either of these foods, they were more likely to cache the food that would not be available next day (Raby *et al.*, 2007). As Mendl and Paul (2008) conclude, such work provides strong evidence for the birds having detailed and useable concepts of the future. There must be a range in the complexity of concepts about the future in non-human animals, as stated by Raby and Clayton (2009), some concepts being relatively simple components of body-state control mechanisms in a changing environment, while others involve envisaging future situations, with or without potential impact on the subject individual.

6.6   Concept of Self

A kind of awareness that has been given much attention is to be self-referent and to discriminate labels of self from labels of non-self, a distinction made by Hauber and Sherman (2001) who described the ability as different from being self-aware. Bekoff and Sherman (2004) said that self-awareness is the cognitive process that enables an individual to discriminate between its own body or possessions and those of others. However, as Broom (2010a) points out, this is a description of a consequence rather than a definition. An individual could be self-aware in the absence of any cue from others. The inclusion of possessions in the description of self-awareness by Bekoff and Sherman is of particular interest. It means that a dog that defends its own bone, but does not defend the bone of another dog, could be called self-aware. Similarly, according to the Bekoff and Sherman statement, a bird that defends its territory but not an adjacent area could also be called self-aware. Most people would say that neither of these capabilities involves self-awareness. The definition proposed here is: self-awareness is the cognitive process in an individual when it identifies and has a concept of its body or possessions as being its own so that it can discriminate these from non-self stimuli.

The preoccupation with self-awareness seems to me to be out of proportion to its intrinsic interest. Why should self-knowledge be considered to be so different from knowledge of the external world? An understanding of the complex processes in the detectable world, especially where an individual has sequential interactions with them, modifying responses over time, requires a very high level of awareness. As mentioned in Sections 4.2 and 6.1, dealing with social situations demands much from brain processing. Many studies of behaviour provide evidence of a high degree of awareness of the self in relation to the world around. For example, without self-knowledge, a lion would risk eating its own forepaws when devouring prey and small animals would start fights with large animals (Grind, 1997).

Are animals aware of their own learning or achievement? In the study by Hagen and Broom (2004) mentioned in Section 4.11, the emotional responses of young cattle were monitored during a period when they were learning a task. Heifers were put into a small pen with a gate through which a food bowl could be seen 15 m away (Fig. 6.1). If a heifer put her nose into a hole in the wall and broke a light beam, the gate opened. When the heifers learned how to open the gate, they showed behavioural excitement in the form of jumping and bucking, and an elevated heart-rate response at the moment of learning. Matched control heifers that received the same reward after the same time in the pen did not show this response and neither did heifers that had previously learned the task and immediately opened the gate on entering the test pen. Similar results were obtained by Broom and Barone (in preparation) in a study on sheep learning. It may be that the animals were aware of their own success in solving a problem so the phenomenon was called the 'eureka' effect.

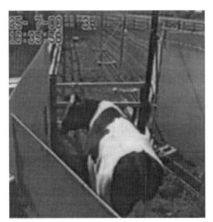 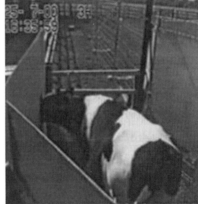

Fig. 6.1. The experimental and control heifers were put in a pen and could see a food bowl at the end of a runway. The two photographs show the experimental heifer (left) putting her nose in the hole in the wall and (right) breaking a beam to make the gate open and give access to the food bowl. The control heifer could not control gate opening. Her gate opened at the time when the other heifer broke the beam, so she was rewarded but did not learn. The excitement response of the experimental heifer when she learned, not shown by the control heifer, is called the 'eureka' effect (photograph K. Hagen).

An individual capable of assessment awareness may be able to learn about what it sees in a mirror in relation to itself and then to use the information at a later time (Broom *et al.*, 2009; Broom, 2010a). The question of whether or not response to a mark seen only in the mirror is evidence for self-awareness is posed by Heyes (1994, 1995) but a substantial degree of awareness is needed to learn what is in a mirror. The studies described in Section 4.6 show how human infants can use mirrors and become aware of what they see. Most young children are told what can be seen in a mirror so it is difficult to establish when they might work this out for themselves. The television studies (see Section 4.6) indicate that awareness of what they see is not apparent until 2–4 years of age. Animals that can learn about what they see in a mirror include chimpanzees, an elephant, dolphins, magpies and pigs. It is likely that such awareness will be demonstrated in other species of animals in future.

A further kind of awareness about self involves being able to think about something that one has in an abstract way. Higher-order thoughts are thoughts about one's own thoughts. These are difficult to demonstrate (but see Section 4.7).

6.7 Awareness of Others Having Concepts

Most discussions of awareness refer to the social context and to whether animals are able to infer the mental states of others (Gallup, 1998). Shettleworth (2009) says that to have a 'theory of mind' means understanding that other individuals have minds. However, I find the term 'mind' imprecise and the distinction between mind and brain unnecessary (Broom, 2003).

Where one individual is aware that another individual has information, it may be possible for us to know this if the first copies what the second does. In the studies of Held *et al.* (2000) (Section 4.6) a pig watched another pig that could see a food location and then did what the other pig had done to get food. A somewhat more complex ability was shown by Miklósi *et al.* (2000) whose dogs demonstrated awareness of another individual having capacity to obtain a resource. The dog saw a toy being hidden in an area that it could not reach. When a human helper arrived, the dog signalled to the helper where the toy was. These dogs must have: (i) had a concept of the position of the object; (ii) remembered this while no human was present; (iii) had a concept of a human having ability to get the object; and (vi) had the ability to link this to the concept that a signal could make a human get the object for the dog. Similar abilities are demonstrated by a dog that responds to a human indicating which object to take. Dogs can do this by using human gaze direction (Reid, 2009) but apes are not good at responding to a human in this way. On the other hand, while apes could track an object hidden in a container when the container was moved, dogs could do this only if the container was moved in a simple way and not if the paths of two similar containers crossed their own path (Rooijakkers *et al.*, 2009).

In a further study with pigs, Held *et al* (2002) described the feeding strategy of a pig that watched an informed but subordinate individual and robbed it when it found food. Subordinate individuals that observed food being hidden by a person, although they went to the food if able to do so, refrained from going to it if a dominant pig were present. These pigs had a concept of the dominant pig taking the food from them if they went to it and hence delayed their action until there was a good chance that they could retain the food. They were aware of the likely consequences of their action and of the behaviour of another animal before it happened.

Actions of animals that use others to obtain objectives are described by Byrne (1997) as Machiavellian. The animals are sufficiently aware of likely events and consequences of actions to be able to manipulate the behaviour of others, maximize the likelihood of benefit and minimize the risk of negative consequences. Another example from pig research by Curtis (1983) is of young pigs that learned to raise or lower environmental temperature by putting the nose in a hole where a light beam was broken. Many of the pigs were able to control the heaters by nudging other pigs to make them switch the heaters on or off. These pigs must have been aware that the other pigs had the capability of remedying adverse temperature conditions. They had the ability to carry out the action needed to change temperature themselves. Hence it is likely that they were aware of what would happen in the near future if they nudged the pig.

6.8   Evolution of Awareness

The genes that promote the capacity to suffer clearly confer an advantage on those individuals that bear them. Hence, to have the extent of awareness needed for suffering is useful. The idea that categories of awareness – or, as Grind and others have put it, 'conscious experiences'– have evolved gradually in number and kind is termed 'gradualism'. An area of awareness that is suggested by Merker (2007) to have evolved is that required to allow sensory arrays to deliver information that changes continuously as a result of self-induced motion. In the evolutionary processes discussed by Grind (2002), the emotional dimension is considered to have been leading the cognitive dimension and there is sometimes mention of pain and other feelings occurring at an early stage.

Motivation and Needs

7

7.1 Motivation

What makes a person, or an animal of any kind, act as they do in any circumstance and at any time? This is a question about the motivation of the individual. Motivation is the process within the brain controlling which behaviours and physiological changes occur, and when. An understanding of motivation is fundamental to all studies of behaviour and is especially relevant to most of the questions asked about human behaviour and about animal behaviour by those managing animals (e.g. concerning feeding, reproduction and handling). An appreciation of the subtleties of motivational systems is also necessary in order that behaviour can be used as an indicator of animal welfare.

At any moment, an individual might initiate an activity because it is likely to result in obtaining food, for example walking to a place where food could be present or starting an action that results in obtaining food that has been detected. A number of factors could affect whether or not these behaviours are shown. There might be sensory input to the brain about the body's environment, including when a food odour is detected or a possible food item is seen. There will be internal input from body monitors, such as those affected by gut distension or blood nutrient levels, which provide information about general or specific body deficiencies. There could be internal input from oscillators within the body that produce an output after a particular time and can indicate normal feeding time or interval since the last feed. Each of these factors has some direct relevance to the feeding system but the likelihood of food-searching will also be affected by inputs to the brain about other aspects of the animal's life. Possibilities include: (i) input about a skin irritation that results in scratching and rubbing rather than food-searching; (ii) input about the presence of a potential mate, rival or source of danger that again leads to some other activity being given priority over food-searching; or (iii) various aspects of hormonal state that change the likelihood of occurrence of the various behaviours.

All of the factors mentioned above, and hence the behaviour initiated, will be altered by the previous experience of that animal. Previous experience that might make an individual less likely to start trying to obtain a food item include: (i) knowing that to take the food would have a negative consequence; (ii) cues that indicate that food provision is imminent; or (iii) information that a higher-priority action is needed. Any input to the decision making centre in the brain must be interpreted in relation to previous experience. Some inputs will never reach the decision making centre in the brain because the interpretation results in their relevance being assessed as zero. It seems likely that most inputs will reach the centre after modification. The inputs to the decision-making centre, following interpretation in the light of experience of a wide variety of external changes and internal states of the body, are called causal factors. At any moment there will be very many different causal factors and the levels of these will determine what the individual actually does. Some causal factor levels will change very rapidly because they are altered by rapidly changing environmental events. Others, such as those that depend upon the levels of certain steroid hormones in the blood, change slowly. All changes in behaviour and some changes in physiological condition are a manifestation of the individual's response to changes in causal factors.

A wide range of causal factors affects the behaviour and physiology of humans and other animals, so motivational state is a combination of all of the levels of all causal factors. Motivational systems have evolved. They enable individuals to ascribe priorities to certain actions, as well as to determine the timing of actions (Broom, 1981a). This facilitates adaptation. For more information on motivation see Toates (2002) or Broom and Fraser (2007). The great importance of the study of motivation in relation to understanding needs and welfare, and the assessment of both of these, is explained below and in Chapter 8.

7.2   Needs

In order that welfare can be good rather than poor, it is important to know the needs of the animal, hence most accounts of the welfare of a particular kind of animal start with a summary of its needs. For example, see the various EFSA Scientific Reports, such as EFSA (2009), and Council of Europe Recommendations, such as Council of Europe (1999). Unsatisfied needs are often (but not always) associated with bad feelings, while satisfied needs may be associated with good feelings. When needs are not satisfied, welfare will be poorer than when they are satisfied.

The motivation system functions to control interactions with the environment, promoting the occurrence of optimal responses and initiation of actions, by means of a set of needs. A need is a requirement, which is part of the basic biology of an animal, to obtain a particular resource or respond to a particular environmental or bodily stimulus (Broom and Johnson, 1993; Broom, 2008a). The need itself is in the brain and allows effective functioning of the animal. It may be fulfilled by physiology or behaviour but the need is not physiological or behavioural.

Some needs are for particular resources, such as water or heat, but control systems have evolved in animals in such a way that the means of obtaining a particular objective have become important to the individual animal (Hughes and Duncan, 1988; Toates and Jensen, 1991; Broom and Johnson, 1993). The animal may need to perform a certain behaviour and may be seriously affected if unable to carry out the activity, even in the presence of the ultimate objective of the activity. For example rats and ostriches will work, in the sense of carrying out actions that result in food presentation, even in the presence of food. In the same way, pigs need to root in soil or some similar substratum (Hutson, 1989), hens need to dust-bathe (Vestergaard, 1980) and both of these species need to build a nest before giving birth or laying eggs (Brantas, 1980; Arey, 1997). In all of these different examples the need itself is in the brain and is not physiological or behavioural, but may be satisfied only when some physiological imbalance is prevented or rectified, or when some particular behaviour is shown.

Needs can be identified by studies of motivation and by assessing the extent of poor welfare in individuals whose needs are not satisfied, and by assessing the extent of good welfare when they are satisfied (Hughes and Duncan, 1988; Dawkins, 1990; Broom and Fraser, 2007). In studies assessing motivational strength (see Chapter 8), the methodology depends on the cognitive ability of the animals (Broom, 2010a).

7.3   Freedoms

The concept of freedom and its relationship to discussions about animal welfare are discussed in Section 2.5. The idea of providing for 'the five freedoms', was first suggested in the Brambell Report in 1965 but it was not quite in line with Thorpe's concept of needs (Brambell *et al.*, 1965; Thorpe, 1965). The list of freedoms just provides a general guideline for non-specialists. Animals have many needs and these have been investigated for many species. Hence the rather general idea of freedoms is now replaced by the more scientific concept of needs. This is the starting point for reviews of the welfare of a species. A list of needs has been the starting point for Council of Europe recommendations and EU scientific reports on animal welfare for over 20 years. The freedoms are not precise enough to be used as a basis for assessment of the welfare of a particular species or group of closely related species.

7.4   Welfare in Relation to Needs

How do we find out from animals what they need? What is preferred? We can ask how hard the individual will work for a resource. For example, in work with rats given a choice of floors, one measure is how often they choose each floor. However, more information is obtained if the rats have to work in order to get to the floor of their choice. A rat can readily learn to lift a weighted door and the amount lifted gives an indication of its strength of preference for the resource (Manser *et al.*, 1996). Sophisticated strength of preference studies depend upon the use of operant and other techniques that exploit the abilities of animals to learn to carry out new procedures (Matthews and Ladewig, 1994; Fraser and Matthews, 1997; Kirkden *et al.*, 2003; see also Chapter 8). Terminology used in motivational strength estimation for an individual includes the following (Kirkden *et al.*, 2003):

- A resource is a commodity or an opportunity to perform an activity.
- The demand is a measured amount of action which enables a resource to be obtained.
- The price is the amount of that action required for a unit of resource.
- The income is the amount of time or other variable limiting that action.
- The price elasticity of demand is the proportional rate at which consumption or demand changes with price.
- The consumer surplus is a measure of the largest amount that a subject is prepared to spend on a given quantity of the resource. It corresponds to an area beneath an inverse demand curve.

An example of the use of this methodology is the work of Mason *et al.* (2001). The key question asked in this work was to ascertain the strength of preference of mink, a partially aquatic species, for various resources, including water in which they could swim. The mink were trained to perform operants to reach: an extra nest, various objects, a raised platform, a tunnel, an empty cage, and a water pool to swim in. The swimming water was given very high priority by the mink.

7.5   Assessing What is Important to Animals

Since aspects of motivational systems have evolved and exist now because they are adaptive, most of the strong preferences of animals are for resources or actions that benefit them: that is, they help them to survive and breed successfully. During development, individuals will have acquired further information that helps them to take decisions that lead to benefits. A consequence of this, pointed out by Duncan (1978, 1992), Dawkins (1983, 1990), Broom and Johnson (1993) and others, is that the assessment of motivational strength during tests of preference is important in any attempt to ensure that poor welfare is avoided and good welfare is maximized in animals kept or affected by man.

It is possible in such, rather laborious, studies to investigate only a few individuals. The variability among animals of a species, and especially the effects of previous living conditions, must be taken into account in interpreting the results. However, it is of great importance to find out what is important to animals of the species studied. Some interesting information about human needs has come from studies of strength of preference studies.

Some studies of preferences have involved observation of what animals choose to do or to obtain when they have a wide variety of opportunities for action. Stolba and Wood-Gush (1989) recorded how sows allocated their time and energy to different behaviours when put in an area of grassland and woodland but were provided with the same concentrate food, in the same quantity, as that given to confined sows. During daylight the sows spent 31% of their time grazing, 21% rooting, 14% in locomotion and only 6% lying. Any preference action requires the animal to make a sacrifice of some sort when it gains access to some quantity of the resource or spends time consuming it. These sows paid a price for carrying out each activity in that they could have done something else instead. Some examples of the many types of preference tests (Fraser and Matthews, 1997; Broom and Fraser, 2007) are described below.

Much of the information that we have about what conditions result in good welfare has been obtained from studies demonstrating positive preferences. What do people choose and what do the animals that we keep choose? If we know this, we have some information about their needs and can provide for them. Ideally, we want to have some quantitative information about the strength of any preference.

An early study of farm animal preferences was that by Hughes and Black (1973) showing that hens given a choice of different kinds of floor to stand on would choose to stand on one of them. In this simple choice test, the cost of choosing involves only the expenditure of the small amount of energy required to move from one floor area to another, so the major sacrifice made when choosing one floor type is not to be standing or lying on another floor type. The choice test is of some value to the animal welfare scientist when comparing resources that satisfy the same or a very similar need. Even in that case, more information is required, because of two resources compared, both may be of low value to the animal or both may be of value but only as luxury items. As Dawkins (1993) explained, a person may choose caviar over smoked salmon, but welfare would not be poor if only one of these were available. Choice tests are of little value where resources associated with different needs, whose motivational basis is quite different, are to be compared (Kirkden et al., 2003). The needs may vary, not only in motivational strength but also in the rate at which they can be satiated or the quantity of the resource required for satiation. Hence more sophisticated preference tests are needed.

One way to assess strength of preference is to balance the preference for a resource of unknown value to the individual with that of a resource whose value is already established. Taking advantage of the fact that gilts preferred to lie in a pen adjacent to other gilts, van Rooijen (1980) offered them the choice of different kinds of floors that were either in pens next to another gilt or in pens further away. With the floor preference titrated against the social preference he was able to get better information about strength of preference. In the work of Arey (1992), the strength of preference was evaluated by measuring how often the subject would press a panel in order to obtain a resource. Preparturient sows would press a panel for access to a room containing straw or one that was empty or containing food. If, in terms of energy and time, it was cheap to get to the straw, the sows opened the door to the straw much more often than the door to the empty compartment. With straw on one side and food on the other, both were chosen if the cost, in terms of number of plate presses required for access, was low. Increasing the ratio of presses to each door opening increased the cost of access and, up to 2 days before parturition, they pressed more often for access to food than for access to straw. At this time, food was more important to the sow than straw for manipulation or nest-building. However, on the day before parturition, at which time a nest would normally be built, sows pressed just as often for straw as for food.

Another indicator of the effort an individual is willing to use to obtain a resource is the weight of a door that has to be lifted. Manser *et al.* (1996), studying floor preferences of laboratory rats, found that rats would lift a heavier door to reach a solid floor on which they could rest than to reach a grid floor. Rats were also found to lift close to the maximum weight possible in order to reach bedding and a dark nest box (Manser *et al.*, 1998a,b).

Welfare Assessment

8

8.1 Positive and Negative Welfare, Short-term and Long-term Assessment

The concept of welfare is explained in Chapter 3, together with its relationships to other concepts. At a particular time, the welfare of an individual may be at any point on a range from very poor to very good. The aim of welfare assessment is to measure how good or how poor the welfare is. Most of this chapter concerns the measures that could be obtained by an animal welfare scientist with a substantial amount of time and the scientific resources to collect them. Some of the measures are readily obtained by less expert persons who have much less time to collect the information than a research scientist would have. Measures that are suitable for relatively brief inspection of animals are described in Section 8.7.

Welfare can be poor because of a specific experience, such as tissue damage and consequent pain, or because of general lack of control over interactions with the environment. Whether people are considering human welfare or the welfare of animals that we keep, there is often more emphasis given to acute painful experiences than to the kind of major problem in life that might lead to depression or other long-lasting abnormalities of brain, behaviour and physiology. Total lack of stimulation, prolonged lack of important stimuli or frequent fear are often much more important causes of poor welfare than temporary pain. Animals, including humans, may suffer greatly as a result of prolonged boredom, frustration or exposure to attacks. The result may be: (i) apathetic behaviour; (ii) abnormalities in behaviour such as stereotypies; (iii) immunosuppression; or (iv) deterioration in brain function.

Is good welfare solely the absence of poor welfare or is it the extent of contentment or pleasure? Most animal welfare scientists would say that it is both (e.g. Würbel, 2009). A review by Boissy *et al.* (2007) concludes that it is a serious mistake to assume that good welfare is just absence of poor welfare.

Welfare indicators are described by Broom and Fraser (2007) and in Section 8.2. Some measurements give information about the welfare at that moment while others indicate welfare during a few seconds, minutes, days or months. There are differences between welfare indicators for short-term and long-term problems. Short-term measures such as heart rate and plasma cortisol concentration are appropriate for assessing welfare during handling or transport but not during long-term housing. Some measures of behaviour, immune system function and disease state are more appropriate for long-term problems. Welfare over longer periods is sometimes referred to as quality of life. This term is much used by clinicians. It means welfare over a period of more than a few days so is quantifiable (Broom, 2007b).

Over any timescale, measures of intensity of effect on welfare have to be related to the duration of the state. When welfare is evaluated, the relationship between its intensity (the word 'severity' is sometimes used where the effect is negative) and duration should be taken into account. Figure 8.1 was initially drawn to exemplify poor welfare during killing methods (Broom, 2001b) but the principle is the same for positive effects.

8.2   Behavioural, Physiological and Clinical Indicators of Poor Welfare

Some welfare indicators are listed in Table 8.1.

8.2.1   Physiological measures

Details of animal welfare assessment are described by Broom and Fraser (2007) and Fraser (2008). Many useful measures are also described in the reports of Welfare Quality (2009 a,b,c).

Some signs of poor welfare arise from physiological measurements. For instance increased heart rate, adrenal activity, or reduced immunological response when a pathogen or other foreign protein is present, can all indicate that welfare is poorer than in individuals which do not show such changes. Care must be taken when interpreting such results, as with many other measures described here.

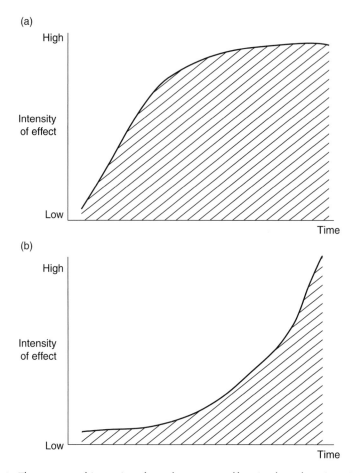

Fig. 8.1. The measured intensity of good or poor welfare is plotted against time for two examples: (a) might be an animal being killed by a method involving prolonged pain and other poor welfare; (b) might be an animal being killed by a method that has a much more rapid effect. The magnitude of good or poor welfare is the area under the curve (modified after Broom, 2001c).

In the case of hypothalamic–pituitary–adrenal (HPA) cortex activity, which leads to increased production of cortisol or corticosterone making more energy available from glycogen reserves, the response may occur because of increased activity level, or excitement associated with courtship or mating. If the objective is to identify the extent of any emergency response, the context of the HPA response must therefore be taken into account. It is usually obvious whether a response is to potential danger or to a sexual partner and it is usually possible to take account of activity levels. If a treatment results in more walking or running, this can be measured and control glucocorticoid responses with such activity level can be used to assess the component of the response that is emergency response.

Table 8.1. Measures of welfare (after Broom and Fraser, 2007).

Physiological indicators of pleasure
Behavioural indicators of pleasure
Extent to which strongly preferred behaviours can be shown
Variety of normal behaviours shown or suppressed
Extent to which normal physiological processes and anatomical development are
   possible
Extent of behavioural aversion shown
Physiological attempts to cope
Immunosuppression
Disease prevalence
Behavioural attempts to cope
Behaviour pathology
Brain changes
Body damage prevalence
Reduced ability to grow or breed
Reduced life expectancy

The glucocorticoid cortisol is produced by the HPA axis in mammals such as Primates, Carnivora and Ungulata; in many fish; and in other animals. Corticosterone has the same function, in particular in rodents and many birds, including poultry. Glucocorticoids have other important functions. There is a daily fluctuation in plasma cortisol concentration and this is associated with the facilitation of effective learning via the functioning of the hippocampus in the brain and maintenance of other normal functions in the body (Broom and Zanella, 2004).

Measurements of glucocorticoids in plasma and saliva are of particular use in studies of the welfare of animals during short-term management practices. If a dog or cat is handled or treated by a veterinary surgeon, the magnitude of the coping response of the animal can be usefully estimated by comparing cortisol concentration in handled and control individuals. When animals are transported, the effects of the various components of the transport process can be assessed by monitoring glucocorticoid concentrations. In all of such studies, the effects of the sampling procedure itself on the animal must be assessed. Since the time to the increase in cortisol concentration is usually 1.5–3 min, the true response is seen if samples can be taken quickly. If samples can be taken with minimal disturbance of the animal, the coping response can be evaluated effectively.

An example of a circumstance in which cortisol measurement gave useful information is the study of Parrott *et al.* (1998) on the effects of loading and transport on the welfare of sheep. The sheep showed a very marked increase in plasma cortisol when they were loaded onto the vehicle. This occurred despite the fact that the staff concerned were experienced animal handlers and did not treat the animals roughly. The sheep were clearly very disturbed by the loading and the response lasted for 6 h. The cortisol concentration then dropped to close to the basal level as the sheep became accustomed to their new environment. During the last 3 h of the journey, the cornering and accelerations caused problems for the sheep, so cortisol concentration increased. These substantial responses of the animal to loading and to the vehicle movements on a winding road were not readily measureable using other indicators. Where it is not easy to take a sample of blood or saliva, HPA axis activity can be assessed by measuring glucocorticoids or their metabolites in urine or faeces. The time for the excreted substances to get into the urine or faeces must be taken into account.

Glucocorticoid measurements are of less use when housing or other long-term treatment is being evaluated because the response adapts after some minutes or hours. Multiple activation of the HPA axis can sometimes lead to measurements of elevation in cortisol over a period of some days. However, lack of increase in glucocorticoids over long periods in a particular housing condition or other treatment does not mean that the welfare is good. For example, severe chronic pain, an ambient temperature above the readily tolerable range and close confinement that allows little movement are not usually associated with elevated cortisol. Other indicators of welfare are needed in these circumstances. Increased glucocorticoid production may lead to immunosuppression. The impaired immune system function and some of the physiological changes can indicate what has been termed a pre-pathological state (Moberg, 1985).

The heart rate of animals changes according to activity and perceived need for activity. The response is relatively rapid and brief, often adapting in 1–2 min. If a cat stands up from a lying position, starts walking, then starts running, its heart rate will increase with each of these activity changes. Were the cat to detect imminent danger at any stage during these changes, a further increase in heart rate would be superimposed. Heart rate can be a useful indicator of short-term welfare problems. In order to evaluate the component of the heart-rate change that is a response to the problem encountered by the individual, the activity level of that individual should be taken into account. An example of a study in which this was done is the work of Baldock and Sibly (1990) who recorded sheep heart rate during different activities and hence were able to assess the magnitude of responses to stimuli presented to the animals. These sheep, which were accustomed to frequent human contact, showed almost maximal heart-rate increase when approached by a dog. It is clear that dogs are very frightening to sheep. Heat stress in livestock results in changes in several physiological and behavioural measures (Phillips and Santurtun, 2013).

A variety of other measurements can be used when attempting to assess the welfare of animals during transport or other relatively short-term treatments. A summary of such measurements is shown in Table 8.2, where most of the substance concentrations were measured in blood but sometimes in other body fluids. If transport is prolonged, food deprivation and rapid metabolism can lead to the metabolism of: (i) food reserves; and then (ii) functional body tissues. The metabolites of each can be identified and measured. Dehydration, bruising, fear, distress, motion sickness and attempts to combat pathogens also lead to recognizable physiological changes.

Table 8.2. Physiological indicators of welfare: short-term problems (modified after Broom and Fraser, 2007).

Stressor	Physiological variable
Food deprivation	↑ FFA, ↑ β-OHB, ↓ glucose, ↑ urea
Dehydration	↑ Osmolality, ↑ total protein, ↑ albumin, ↑ PCV
Physical exertion, bruising	↑ CK, ↑ LDH5,↑ lactate
Fear	↑ Cortisol, ↑ PCV, ↑ heart rate, ↓ heart-rate variability, ↑ respiration rate, ↑ LDH5
Motion sickness	↑ Vasopressin
Inflammation, large immunological responses	↑ Acute phase proteins, e.g. haptoglobin, C-reactive protein, serum amyloid-A
Hypothermia/hyperthermia	Change in body and skin temperature, ↑ prolactin

FFA, free fatty acids; β-OHB, beta-hydroxy butyrate; PCV, packed cell volume; CK, creatine kinase; LDH5, lactate dehydrogenase isoenzyme 5.

8.2.2   Behavioural measures

Behavioural measures are of particular value in welfare assessment. If an individual avoids an object or event strongly, this behaviour gives information about its feelings and about its welfare. When an object is present or an event is occurring, the greater the efforts made to avoid, the worse the welfare that is indicated. Another behavioural measure is whether or not a behaviour that the animal is strongly motivated to show can be carried out. An individual that is completely unable to adopt a preferred lying posture, despite repeated attempts, will be assessed as having poorer welfare than one which can adopt the preferred posture. Other abnormal behaviour such as stereotypies, self-mutilation, tail-biting in pigs, feather-pecking in hens or excessively aggressive behaviour indicate that the perpetrator's welfare is poor.

Stereotypies and other abnormal behaviours are used as welfare indicators (see Chapters 23–27 of Broom and Fraser, 2007). A stereotypy is a repeated, relatively invariate sequence of movements which has no obvious function. For example, some sows confined in stalls or tethers may spend many hours showing stereotypies such as that shown in Fig. 8.2, repeatedly pressing the drinker without drinking. The sequence of events recorded using video for such a sow was repeated very many times. Other examples of stereotypies include tail-chasing in dogs and crib-biting and tongue-drawing in horses. Locomotor stereotypies are not normal, generally rewarding movements such as walking or running, where these have an objective (e.g. getting to a place or exercising) but are those movements without such a function (e.g. the route-tracing of some zoo animals or of people in solitary confinement). All stereotypies tend to occur in circumstances where the individual lacks control over its interactions with its environment, and they indicate poor welfare. Environmental enrichment can reduce the extent of poor welfare and the occurrence of stereotypies (Mason et al., 2007).

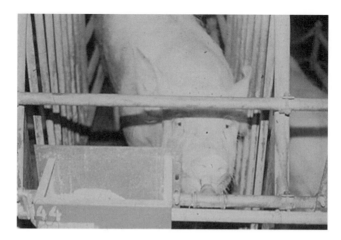

Fig. 8.2. A pregnant sow, confined in a stall, showing a drinker-pressing stereotypy (photograph D.M. Broom, from Broom and Fraser, 2007).

Other abnormal behaviours that can be quantified and used as indicators of long-term welfare problems include excessively aggressive behaviour and inactive unresponsive behaviour. Excessive aggression is often thought of as a fault that the individual should prevent. Although feelings of aggression can often be curbed, and it is advantageous to do so in order to retain a position in a social group, aggressive behaviour can also be a consequence of a major inadequacy in the individual's environment. Aggression can indicate poor welfare in the aggressive individual, as well as causing it in others, in humans and in other animals. In humans, inactivity and lack of responses to stimuli that would normally elicit a response are used as indicators of depression. Close confinement and inability to avoid being attacked or otherwise harmed may well lead to behavioural signs of depression in a range of captive animals.

When there are either physiological or behavioural responses to adversity, in some cases it is clear that the individual is trying to cope with adversity, and the extent of the attempts to cope can be measured. In other cases, however, the responses are solely pathological and the individual is failing to cope. In either circumstance the measure indicates poor welfare.

A further general method of welfare assessment listed in Table 8.1 involves measuring what behaviour and other functions cannot be carried out in particular living conditions. Hens prefer to flap their wings at intervals but cannot in a battery cage; while veal calves and some caged laboratory animals try hard to groom themselves thoroughly but cannot in a small crate, cage or restraining apparatus.

In all welfare assessment it is necessary to take account of individual variation in attempts to cope with adversity and in the effects that adversity has on the animal. When pigs have been confined in stalls or tethers for some time, a proportion of individuals show high levels of stereotypies, while others are very inactive and unresponsive (Broom, 1987). There may also be a change, with time spent in the condition, in the amount and type of abnormal behaviour shown (Cronin and Wiepkema, 1984). In rats, mice and tree shrews it is known that individuals confined with an aggressor show different physiological and behavioural responses, categorized as involving active or passive coping (von Holst, 1986; Koolhaas *et al.*, 1999). Active animals fight vigorously whereas passive animals submit. A study of the strategies adopted by gilts in a competitive social situation showed that some sows were aggressive and successful, a second category of animals defended vigorously if attacked, while a third category of sows avoided social confrontation if possible. These categories of animals differed in their adrenal responses and in reproductive success (Mendl *et al.*, 1992). As a result of differences in the extent of different physiological and behavioural responses to problems it is necessary that any assessment of welfare should include a wide range of measures. Our knowledge of how the various measurements combine to indicate the severity of the problem must also be improved.

8.2.3   Disease, injury, movement and growth measures

In addition to behavioural observations, a range of measures that might be obtained during clinical examination of an individual and checking of clinical records can provide important measures of welfare. Disease, injury, movement difficulties and growth abnormality all indicate poor welfare. In comparative investigations of welfare in carefully controlled studies, if the incidence of any of the above is significantly increased, the welfare of the individuals is worse in that system or circumstance. The welfare of any diseased individual is worse than one that is not diseased, but much remains to be discovered about the magnitude of the effects of disease on welfare. We still have much to learn about how much suffering is associated with different diseases. People who report that they are suffering may be given a sedative, anti-inflammatory or analgesic drug, but the information available to the physician is often not very accurate. People report suffering with varying degrees of accuracy, and knowledge of clinical signs or of the expected progression of a diagnosed clinical condition. Hence the reports do not allow precise estimation of the various kinds of suffering.

A specific example in farm animals of an effect on housing conditions that leads to poor welfare is the consequence of severely reduced exercise for bone strength. In studies of hens (Knowles and Broom, 1990; Nørgaard-Nielsen, 1990), birds that could not sufficiently exercise their wings and legs because they were housed in battery cages had considerably weaker bones than birds in percheries where they could and did exercise. Similarly, Marchant and Broom (1996) found that sows in stalls had leg bones only 65% as strong as sows in group-housing systems. The actual weakness of bones means that the animals are coping less well with their environment so welfare is poorer in the confined housing. If such an animal's bones are broken there will be considerable pain and the welfare will be worse. We can reasonably assume that a broken bone leads to pain and other suffering, and examples of evaluation of pain are presented below in Section 8.3.

On most occasions when a clinician is attempting to evaluate the welfare of an individual, the evidence is less clear-cut than a broken, or even a weakened bone. Poor welfare other than that resulting from pain is often not reported systematically in relation to human patients or veterinary patients. However, measures of behaviour, physiology including body fluid biochemistry, extent of bruising or lesions, amount of detectable inflammation of tissue and other indicators can be cross-related to provide more accurate information about the welfare of the individual. This clinical assessment of welfare is a developing area of medical and veterinary science.

8.3   Pain Assessment

The problem that is often stated in relation to pain in species other than man is that the animals cannot tell you when they are in pain or how bad it is. However, the major method used in human pain studies is self-reporting, for example on a scale from no pain to very severe pain. How reliable is this? People can lie or deceive themselves in relation to pain. Our knowledge of pain in non-humans is based on measures of observed behaviour or physiological change. These measures will often be more accurate than those conventionally used during medical evaluation, so should be better developed for humans and in veterinary diagnosis (Broom, 2001b).

Some methods for recognizing and assessing non-human pain have been used for a long time. For example the tail-flick response of rats since 1941, the jaw-opening response since 1964, limb-withdrawal since 1975 and self-mutilation for much longer (Dubner, 1994). Sophisticated behavioural measures are being used more and more in studies of pain. However, there are problems in pain recognition which make comparisons between species difficult. Severe pain can exist without any detectable sign. Individuals within a species vary in the thresholds for the elicitation of pain responses. Most difficult for the general public, as well as for those studying the subject, is that species vary in the kinds of behavioural responses that are elicited by pain (Morton and Griffiths, 1985). Hence it is important to consider which behavioural pain responses are likely to be adaptive for any species under consideration. Humans, in common with other large primates, dogs and pigs, live socially and can help one another when attacked by a predator. Parents may help offspring, and other group members may help individuals who are attacked or otherwise in pain. Hence distress signals such as loud vocalizations are adaptive when pain resulting from an injury is felt. Where the members of a species can very seldom collaborate in defence, for example African antelopes that are subject to attack by lions, leopards, hyenas or hunting dogs, or sheep that are subject to attack by wolves, lynx, leopards or mountain lions, the biological situation is quite different. The predators select apparently weak individuals for attack and vocalizations when injured might well attract predators rather than conferring any benefit. As a result, these animals do not vocalize when injured.

In the mulesing operation, devised by Mr Mules to reduce the likelihood of fly-strike, a sheep is caught by humans and put upside down in a holding frame, has a 15-cm diameter area of skin around the anogenital apertures cut off with a pair of scissors and is then turned over and released. The animal often makes no sound and walks away. Farm staff who carry out this procedure may believe that sheep do not feel pain. However, sheep have all of the normal mammalian pain system and they produce high levels of cortisol and β-endorphin after the mutilation (Shutt *et al.*, 1987). Another example concerns monkeys, which, although normally very noisy, are very quiet when giving birth, a time when they are at increased risk from predators. Their silence does not mean that parturition involves no pain. A knowledge of the selective pressures affecting the species is needed before behavioural responses to pain can be interpreted properly. Having explained the difficulties of using behavioural measures of pain, however, there are many examples of studies in which quantitative measurement of pain has been carried out and these are reported in later chapters. A dog or pig in pain will often vocalize, and the pitch and loudness of the sound can be measured. A rat will change its behaviour in several ways, including changes in the amount of locomotion and adopting recognizable postures, all of which can be quantified (Flecknell, 2001).

Behavioural responses to stimuli that would be expected to be painful have been studied in many vertebrates. For example, Verheijen and Buwalda (1988) stimulated the mouth of a carp electrically and recorded fin movements, bradycardia, freezing and erratic darting movements that resulted in collisions with the glass wall of the tank. When studying carp that were hooked in the mouth, Beukema (1970) and Verheijen and Buwalda (1988) measured avoidance of bait. Avoidance learning is reported for fish, for example by Brookshire and Hoegnander (1968) who administered a shock to paradise fish when they entered a black compartment and found that the fish avoided the black compartment subsequently and learned to activate an escape hatch to avoid further shocks.

Opioids have many functions, one of which is natural analgesia. Hence it is of interest to measure concentration changes in encephalins, endorphins and their precursor pro-opiomelanocortin. Behavioural changes may be measured when opioids or opioid receptor inhibitors are injected.

Facial changes during pain are well known in humans but have also been reported for several other mammalian species. Mice show facial changes when they are subjected to treatment that we should normally expect to involve pain (Leach *et al.*, 2012). Studies of horses and sheep also show that painful experiences are reflected in facial changes. The extent of eye-opening, defined by the amount of the white sclera visible, the exact position of the ears and the position of the various parts of the face, as a consequence of movements of facial muscles, can be described (Figs 8.3 and 8.4).

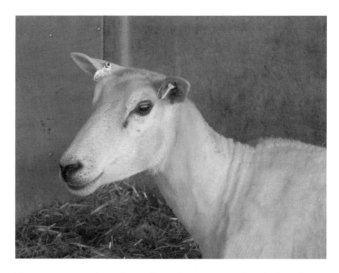

Fig. 8.3. This ewe was not in pain and can be compared with that shown in Fig. 8.4 (photograph K.M. McLennan).

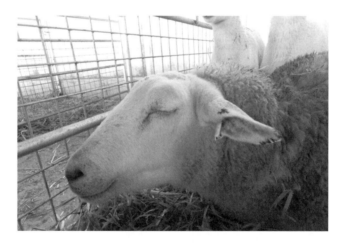

Fig. 8.4. This ewe is showing indicators of extreme pain. She has her eyes clenched shut, her ears pulled back and down, her lower jaw pulled back, and the back of her nostril appears square. She has severe mastitis, infection with *Mannheimia haemolytica* and *Pasteurella trehalosi*, and would not eat or drink. She died a few hours after this photograph was taken (photograph K.M. McLennan; veterinary information courtesy of C.B. Rebelo).

Given the low level of behavioural response when sheep are injured by a predator (and the term 'predator' would include humans) it is of interest to ask how it might be that facial changes during pain occur and have evolved in sheep. One possibility is that the contraction of a muscle, or set of muscles, in an area remote from the pain might reduce the attention paid to the painful area.

A second is that the facial change associated with an injury might deter other social group members from coming close and exacerbating the problem, for example by jostling the affected animal and increasing foot pain. A third possibility could occur if the facial movement is associated with disease, in which case other group members might benefit from not approaching close to the animal in pain.

8.4 Indicators of Good Welfare Including Pleasure, Happiness, Good Health

8.4.1 Reporting on happiness, or direct measurement?

The most widely used argument that the welfare of a person is good is that the person reports that he is happy. In many cases, the person making such a report is correctly describing his state but in some cases he is not. Observation of the person's behaviour, including expression and the extent to which normal activities are carried out, is more likely to give accurate information about how good the individual's welfare is. Other measurements mentioned below can occasionally be used.

8.4.2 Using information about preferences

We already know a lot, in general terms, about human positive and negative preferences. If a person has been forced to stay for a long period in adverse temperature conditions, or has been subject to frightening experiences, or has been kept in close confinement, we expect that her welfare will be poor. If the recent experiences of the individual have been interesting, socially supportive and of a kind that is normally pleasurable, the welfare of the person would be expected to be good. For other animals, if we have the kind of information described in Section 7.5, and hence we know that positive preferences have been fulfilled and negative preferences avoided, we should expect the welfare of those animals to be good. Much of our information about good welfare of humans and non-humans is obtained in this way. However, there are also direct measures of good welfare that can be used.

Several of the tests described in Chapters 4 and 5, such as state-specific conditioning and cognitive bias, can provide information about how good welfare is as well as how poor. Some of the current and potential methodologies are described by Mendl and Paul (2004).

8.4.3 Play and normal behaviour

When they are happy, people and many other species of animals are more likely to play. One form of play is to attempt to carry out an efficient movement but in the absence of the usual objective of the movement. For example, we refer to a kitten chasing a ball as playing, when the chasing movements are those that might be used in later life for catching prey. Active physical play is commoner in young animals and must often help the individual to develop movements that are effective in attaining objectives when older. Since play is thought of as an especially juvenile activity there is reluctance among adults to say that they play.

However, many adult behaviours could also be called play. Adult humans engage in play but it is more often intellectual than physical. There can be play with thoughts or ideas. This may involve no movement or, as in activities such as crossword puzzles or Sudoku, have only a small physical component. Many adult activities, such as leisure reading or conversation over drinks or meals, include an element of play. Indeed it might be said that much academic research is partly play.

One kind of play may be called a game and Suits (1967, 2005) argued that a game is an activity in which we voluntarily choose an inefficient means of achieving a goal so that we can engage in the activity. This does describe some play and games. However, it is not a general definition of games because the term 'game' is also used for contests in which partaking is not voluntary and failure may mean not reproducing, or dying. These contests would not be called play. It would seem that play is carrying out a movement or intellectual process, either in the absence of its usual objective, or by using an inefficient means of achieving a goal solely in order to engage in that movement or process.

Since play occurs in situations when welfare is good, and is generally suppressed when welfare is poor (Boissy *et al.*, 2007), the measurement of play has been proposed as an indicator of good welfare (Held and Spinka, 2011). While most of the behaviour that might be categorized as play is likely to indicate that welfare is good, some intellectual play is not readily identified by observers and some behaviour is not unambiguously play. For example, social play in piglets and other young animals can end in a fight.

Pruitt *et al.* (2011) reported that before mating, the spider *Anelosimus studiosus* showed repeated behaviour that could be regarded as practice or play, and that the spiders that showed play were more successful at mating as a consequence. Since play is often taken to imply a positive feeling in the mammalian literature, did these spiders have positive feelings?

It is often stated that being able to show normal behaviour is a prerequisite for good welfare (see Chapter 5 and Table 8.1). However, behaviour that occurs normally in natural or captive conditions includes responses to predators, pathology and starvation, and these indicate poor welfare. The needs of the individual are a consequence of biological mechanisms and their fulfilment is associated with good welfare. The behaviour shown when all needs are fulfilled would be called normal, so it is having the opportunity to show normal behaviour that can be equated with good welfare. When behaviour is described as abnormal, it is maladaptive and hence associated with some welfare problem. If an individual is not showing abnormal behaviour and has the possibility to carry out any adaptive behaviour that it chooses, welfare is better than in circumstances in which adaptive behaviours cannot be performed. A maladaptive or abnormal behaviour is one that differs in pattern, frequency or context from that which is shown by most members of the species under conditions that would allow a full behavioural range (Broom and Johnson, 1993). For species in captivity, including farm, companion, working, laboratory and zoo animals, it is necessary to carry out careful investigations to determine what is normal behaviour, as they often face environmental challenges that their species will not have encountered during most of their evolution (Knierim *et al.*, 2001; Hill and Broom, 2009). As these authors explain, research of this kind on the needs of the animals requires a thorough knowledge of the biology of the species, but does not necessarily have to be carried out in wild conditions.

8.4.4   Direct measures of good welfare

When a positive event, perhaps a reward, is expected, anticipatory behaviour may occur. Such behaviour is normally easy to distinguish from behaviour in anticipation of a negative event. A variety of behaviours may occur in such circumstances. Hence, movements such as tail-wagging in dogs and expressions such as smiling are often indicators of good welfare. However, they have to be interpreted taking account of the context. Dogs may wag their tails in the presence of a dominant individual (canine or human) who may attack them, so the tail-wag does not always indicate good welfare. Smiling might be forced, although people are usually quite good at detecting this, so genuine smiling is a fairly reliable indicator of good welfare.

Physiological changes in the brain seem to be associated with good welfare on some occasions (Broom and Zanella, 2004). When people were shown happy pictures there was an increase in magnetic resonance imaging (MRI) activity on one side of the frontal area of the cerebral cortex, and amygdala activity dropped. Phillips *et al.* (1998) showed sad pictures to people and scanned their brains using MRI. A set of regions were found in which there was activity during sad but not during neutral or cheerful situations.

As described in Chapter 5, oxytocin is produced in circumstances where there are positive feelings. One such circumstance in a female mammal is nursing the young. Oxytocin is not only associated with the let-down of milk but leads to a feeling of pleasure as well. Oxytocin is synthesized in the paraventricular nucleus (PVN) of the hypothalamus and in the supraoptic nucleus. It binds to receptors that regulate HPA axis activity and its increase is associated with adrenocorticotrophic hormone (ACTH) and glucocorticoid decrease, lymphocyte proliferation, brain gamma-amino butyric acid (GABA) increase and cardiac vagal tone increase (Carter and Altemus, 1997; Redwine *et al.*, 2001; Altemus *et al.*, 2001). In some contexts there is no doubt that good welfare is indicated when oxytocin concentration in the blood increases. There is still a need for more information in order to be sure that there are no negative situations where an increase in oxytocin occurs, but at present the measure looks useful. Change in cardiac vagal tone is another physiological measure that has been used as an indicator of good welfare. In the study of Gygax *et al.* (2013), measurements of prefrontal cortex activity, sympatho-vagal reaction, locomotion and behaviour indicating anticipation near the food bowl were all different in rewarded and frustrated goats.

8.5   Integration of Welfare Measures

When the welfare of a collection of individuals is assessed, sets of measures often have to be integrated: for example, physiological measures, behavioural and pathological measures. While a single measure can indicate poor welfare, because of the variety of coping mechanisms used by individuals and the diversity of consequences of environmental impact, a range of measures will provide better information about welfare.

In scientific studies of animal welfare, a variety of indices should be examined together, including behaviour patterns, frequencies and contexts as well as physiological and other measures. However, during studies of the welfare of zoo animals (Hill and Broom, 2010) and some other captive animals, it may not be possible to utilize a wide range of quantitative measures. Hence some welfare scientists are using a combination of qualitative and quantitative measures in their assessments (Wemelsfelder *et al.*, 2000; Rousing and Wemelsfelder, 2006; Napolitano *et al.*, 2008). Francoise Wemelsfelder argues that people who are familiar with animals of a particular species are able to use a range of obvious and subtle cues to evaluate their welfare, sometimes without knowing what observations they are making to do this. She points out that conclusions based on observation of all of the animal's expression of its current state will reduce the risks of error associated with conclusions based on the recording of single movements. The qualitative behavioural assessment that can be produced is clearly useful in certain circumstances but Wemelsfelder argues that it should be combined with other measures.

The first stage of qualitative behavioural assessment should be careful planning of how the assessment will be conducted. There could be a systematic bias of observers who have preconceived ideas about the effects of the environment or treatment on the animals (Wemelsfelder *et al.*, 2009; Tuyttens *et al.*, 2014). The evaluations of the welfare of the same animal by several people sometimes agree closely. However, during the use of qualitative behavioural assessment, there can be a risk that observers will not use the same observations, and in particular the same weighting of observations, and hence that there could be poor inter-observer reliability. While all measurement is subject to some degree of lack of inter-observer reliability, this risk may be higher when less precisely defined measures are used. In studies such as that of Rousing and Wemelsfelder (2006) the training led to quite good inter-observer reliability. However, in the study of Bokkers *et al.* (2012) the inter-observer reliability was too low for the data to be used. In practice, it is difficult to know whether or not the data reliability is sufficiently good, so when should this methodology be used? It is valuable in some studies where non-scientists are asked to evaluate the welfare of animals and in preliminary studies of work by animal welfare scientists where welfare assessment is proposed. After both of these studies have been undertaken, an investigation of what actual observations were being made can be carried out in order to develop better indicators. In studies by animal welfare scientists, established welfare measures should be used wherever possible and qualitative behavioural assessment should only be used if there is no potential for bias and if inter-observer reliability has been shown to be good.

8.6   Risk and Benefit Analysis in Animal Welfare

The risks that a toxic substance will be in a foodstuff, that a pathogen will enter an animal and proliferate in it, or that a management procedure will result in poor welfare in a farm animal, have always been considered in scientific reports such as those produced by the European Food Safety Authority (EFSA) or its predecessors in the EU and in other countries. However, in recent years the methodology for assessing risk has become more sophisticated and systematic, so it is now used in many scientific reports requested by governments. This has resulted in scientists being more rigorous in their analyses of potential problems. If a quantitative or qualitative risk analysis is carried out, it is less likely that factors that affect the harm under consideration will be missed. Also, the relative importance of the factors involved will often be estimated more accurately. This approach was stimulated by the initial failures in the late 1980s and early 1990s to properly evaluate the risks associated with the outbreak of bovine spongiform encephalopathy (BSE) in cattle and Creutzfeldt–Jakob Disease (CJD) in humans who had consumed some cattle products. A reluctance to harm the cattle and cattle-feed industries led to inadequate analysis of risk to cattle and humans. This might have resulted in the deaths of millions of people. Although new variant CJD (nvCJD) takes a long time to develop in humans, it is already clear that, fortunately, the number of deaths will be very much lower than this. Harm to people and harm to industry is less if a proper risk analysis is conducted at an early stage.

The sequence of procedures during the analysis of risks or benefits is: (i) list factors (hazards if negative); (ii) calculate exposure; (iii) estimate uncertainty. The analysis may be quantitative, if sufficient numerical information is available, or qualitative if it is not. The inclusion of risk analysis in scientific reports and opinions produced by EFSA and other organizations has helped decision makers to take appropriate action: for example, to minimize animal disease and improve animal welfare. It is desirable that this approach should be continued, with suitable modification according to the limitations associated with the relevant data.

Some factors that affect animals have beneficial effects rather than leading to a greater risk of a harm. This is most obvious when the wide-ranging components of animal welfare are considered. Food, access to other resources, human contact, social interactions and many other factors can result in benefit to the individual. Any one of these factors may also stimulate the immune system of an animal and hence confer benefit by reducing the likelihood of clinical disease. Hence every scientific review of welfare in general or of a component of health, such as the occurrence and effects of a pathological condition, should consider the possible beneficial effects of factors as well as their impact on risk. It is not sufficient in such reports to merely conduct a risk analysis.

The first EU scientific reports on animal welfare in which formal risk assessments were carried out were EFSA (2006a,b) 'The risks of poor welfare in intensive calf farming systems' and 'Animal health and welfare risks associated with the import of wild birds, other than poultry, into the European Union'. Since that time, many EFSA reports on animal welfare topics, as well as those on animal disease topics, have included a risk assessment (see Berthe *et al.*, 2012, for further details). A guidance to methods of conducting such risk assessments (EFSA, 2012c) has been produced. Risk assessments have also been conducted outside the EU; see for example Paton and Martin (2006).

8.7   Welfare Reports and Welfare Outcome Indicators for Use in Inspection

When scientific reports on animal welfare matters are produced, these are easier for legislators and other informed persons to use and have greater effect if the primary scientific literature is quoted giving full references (Broom, 2014). However, evaluation of the quality of the scientific information is also important. The conclusions from the data reviewed should be quoted, and recommendations made should be based on the evidence available. Where there is little scientific information, conclusions and recommendations should still be made, but the quality of the information upon which they are based should be made clear. In some cases, it is valid to use information from related species, but in other cases it is not. For example, every social animal will be adversely affected by being tied up and prevented from showing social as well as normal maintenance behaviour, so a report on a social animal that has not been studied directly in this respect could refer to studies of other species. On the other hand, a pathogen that causes infection in one species may not cause infection in another, so extrapolation from species to species is not always reliable.

Some of the causes of animal welfare problems in animals kept for human use are a result of genetic selection while others are a consequence of housing conditions, management methods or procedures used. In order to legislate about such matters, particular practices or systems might be prohibited. However, sometimes bad management in a good system has similar effects on welfare to good management in a less good system, and even the best housing and management may result in poor welfare if the genetic selection is causing the problems. Hence the best way of designing laws may be to require that very negative consequences for animals do not occur, or to ensure that specified good welfare does occur.

Measures used to predict or assess welfare that might be used in laws or codes of practice may include resource-based, management-based or welfare outcome indicators that are animal-based. As an example of the latter, because lameness in broiler chickens and dairy cows is a problem, it is possible to monitor the number of animals that are lame as a welfare outcome indicator. This involves using an animal-based measure. The welfare outcome scored is the animal's ability to walk and this is done using a scientifically designed scale of walking ability. Animals on farm or arriving at a slaughterhouse can be checked and a threshold level of lameness can be used to decide whether or not their welfare complies with the law or code of practice. For example, for dairy cows, the EFSA report and opinions on the welfare of dairy cows (EFSA, 2009) proposed that the threshold for a group of dairy cows on farm or at the slaughterhouse might be 10%. In order to facilitate this approach, EFSA has produced a series of reports and opinions on animal-based welfare outcome indicators for several farm species (EFSA, 2012b,d,e).

The links between factors that might affect welfare and their consequences, which might be used as measures, need to be validated (see EFSA, 2012a). Some are very clear: for example, a bitten pig's tail is easily recognizable. Others are clearly negative: for example, frequent stereotypies indicate substantial problems. However, for other measures the links are less clear: for example, various factors may affect the ratio of heterophil to lymphocyte white blood cells in the blood. A further example, also mentioned in Subsection 8.2.1, is that many causes of poor welfare do not increase cortisol, so absence of cortisol increase does not mean that the individuals have no problems.

Sentience During Development, Brain Damage and Old Age

9

9.1 Introduction: Pre- and Post-sentience

The majority of this book concerns humans and other animals that are free-living, in that they have the physical and mental capability to move around and interact with their environments. There is variation within any species in abilities, as mentioned in earlier chapters, so it is the average individual, or the outstandingly able individual, that is the main subject of discussion. However, when human cognitive and other abilities are compared with those of other species, conclusions have to be qualified in relation to the very young and some of the injured or old. A human child at birth may have the potential to carry out impressive cognitive tasks but has, at that time of life, far less actual ability than many other animals have. A person who has suffered substantial brain damage after an accident, or a person with advanced senile dementia, may be much less able than the pet dog in the same family or the magpie in the garden.

The concept of sentience in relation to embryos, fetuses, newborn or newly hatched individuals is also relevant to ethical decisions about abortion, killing young at birth or hatching and the use of anaesthetics and analgesics for fetuses and very young individuals (see Section 10.5). The evidence about sentience that is relevant to decisions about euthanasia and other humane killing of brain-damaged individuals, or of those whose brain function is substantially impaired because of pathological changes, is discussed here. The ethical decisions are discussed in Section 10.6.

9.2   Sentience in Embryos and Fetuses

9.2.1   Some developmental differences

In this section the point of development at which fetuses and embryos are sentient is considered (EFSA, 2005). It is helpful to distinguish species according to whether they are altricial or precocial at birth. An example of a precocial species is the horse, which is well developed physiologically and behaviourally at birth. Altricial species include marsupials, where the joeys are born at a very early stage of development, and rats, that are a little more developed. There is a gradation between these extremes and humans are altricial but better developed at birth than rats (Broom, 1981b). In birds, many duck species are precocial and show strong following behaviour within minutes of hatching, whereas raptors have a relatively long fledging period before they are able to perform well-coordinated walking or flying. Precocial species depend on greater development and use of sensory faculties from the moment of birth or hatching, whereas this requirement is at a lower level in altricial species.

The differences between oviparous and viviparous species require consideration. The mothers of mammals and other viviparous species could have substantial problems if the fetus or fetuses were too active. A system for the suppression of activity is therefore adaptive in these animals. There could be suppression of consciousness until independent living occurs, usually identified as the time of the onset of breathing. However, there may be advantages associated with an ability to respond to and learn from stimuli received *in utero*, and this could require some degree of awareness. Development in an egg, on the other hand, has less constraint on the development of brain function because movement is physically limited by the eggshell and fetal activity is less risky than it would be in viviparous species. A consequence is that awareness in oviparous species can safely develop earlier and be continuous instead of intermittent. If awareness is the criterion for protection, it may be, therefore, that birds, reptiles, amphibians, fish and cephalopods are more in need of protection pre-hatching than mammals are in need of protection pre-partum.

Shortly after birth, precocial species are able to stand, walk and run. These activities have to be suppressed while the fetus is in the uterus, otherwise they could jeopardize the comfort of the dam, and when violent they could pose a risk of uterine rupture, placental abruption and abortion. Under normal conditions *in utero*, these activities are suppressed through control over fetal oxygenation. Oxygenation in the fetus is normally lower than that in the newborn. If oxygenation is raised artificially, the fetus becomes physically aroused and more active. The situation may, however, be more complex in the case of oviparous species. Some chicks show responses to sounds, touch and light several days before hatching, breathe for many hours before hatching, and there is clicking communication among unhatched chicks ('pipping') which allows synchronization of hatching in some species (Vince, 1973). It may also be that some reptiles develop brain function hours or days before hatching.

While most of the data presented in the text which follows concerns mammals, precocial birds and reptiles have many similarities to precocial mammals in development of potential for awareness, and altricial mammals have similarities to altricial birds. Most amphibians and fish have larval forms that are not well developed at hatching but develop rapidly with experience of independent life. Those fish and amphibians that are well developed at hatching or viviparous birth and all cephalopods (since these are small but well developed at hatching) will have had a functioning nervous system and the potential for awareness for some time before hatching.

9.2.2   Neural and pain system development

Brain development starts long before birth in humans and other mammals. In humans, the number of neurons in the striate cortex, for example, is approximately the same at 28 weeks as it is at 37 weeks, the time of birth, or 3 years, although there are changes in the brain as synaptic density in the visual cortex increases fivefold from 28 weeks to 6 months (Huttenlocher, 1993). Visual tracking and recognition develop between birth and 6 months in human babies (Johnson, 1993) but none of these results mean that some systems do not function earlier in development. In mammalian species such as the human and the rat, sensory pathways in the peripheral nervous system and spinal cord are well developed by the time the individual is born (Anand and Hickey, 1987; Fitzgerald, 1999). They possess the necessary neural structures, neural connections and neurotransmitters for afferent sensory and efferent motor activity that serve a range of functions. In the near-term human fetus there is, however, a limited repertoire of physical movements before birth even though some fetal limb movements may start after 4–5 months of pregnancy. Those movements that do occur are in cycles, usually once every 1–10 min, and limb movements predominate. The activity cycles are similar to those seen in the supine newborn baby, and in the latter they can occur while the baby is asleep as well as awake (Robertson, 1987).

Sensory and neural development in a precocial bird such as the domestic chick is very well advanced several days before hatching. In domestic fowl, hatching occurs after 21 days of incubation. Controlled movements and evoked responses (i.e. coordinated behaviour and electrophysiological change to tactile, auditory and visual stimuli) appear 3–4 days before hatching (Broom, 1981b).

The near-term rat fetus is capable of physical reflex responses to noxious cutaneous stimuli, such as pricking a foot with a needle. The responses are generalized whole-body movements, rather than the typical limb withdrawal response seen later in the infant pup. The transition from generalized to localized types of response is thought to depend on post-natal maturation of central nervous system pathways and the emergence of descending inhibitory control of the generalized writhing movements. The pattern of the prenatal generalized responses is often unpredictable, and this has led observers to suspect that the responses are poorly organized centrally. The onset of transition from generalized to localized responses to potentially painful stimuli may vary between species.

Evidence on the maturity at birth of afferent nociceptive pathways and the central nervous system gives contrasting impressions. The central nervous system in the human fetus is usually considered as being both structurally and functionally immature at the time of birth (Marsh *et al.*, 1997). The term 'immature', however, might mean 'largely functional', even if not in final form. Fetal pain perception is thought to be unlikely before the third trimester (Lee *et al.*, 2005). Not only is there poor central organization in the physical responses to potentially painful stimuli, but there is incomplete development of the afferent activity of the unmyelinated C fibres, which are an important type of nerve fibre for nociception. Taken together, this indicates that opportunities for perceiving some painful stimuli in the fetus are reduced. However, there are other features that suggest the opposite. For example, the exaggerated N-methyl-D-aspartate- (NMDA-)induced responses in the substantia gelatinosa, and the reduced descending inhibition along the spinal cord, imply a capacity for heightened afferent activation of nociceptive pathways. When needles were stuck into human fetuses, they showed increases in plasma cortisol concentrations (Giannakoulopoulos *et al.*, 1994).

The newborn lamb, foal and calf are, in comparison with the rat and human newborn, relatively well developed neurologically and behaviourally. Neural development is sufficiently advanced at full term in the sheep fetus to allow this species to be used as a model for assessing high levels of risk of perception and suffering before and during delivery. This is fortunate, as the sheep has been the preferred species for experimental research into fetal physiology. Corresponding knowledge on arousal is relatively advanced in the sheep fetus.

9.2.3   Awareness in the fetus

The term 'embryo' is used for the unborn offspring from the zygote until all major structures are represented and it is called a fetus after this. Experimental work on conscious awareness in the sheep fetus has been reviewed (Mellor and Gregory, 2003; Lyche *et al.*, 2005; Mellor *et al.*, 2005). In summary, the work indicates that wakefulness does not occur in the fetus until it breathes air after it has been delivered by natural birth or removed from the womb during the latter stages of development when breathing is possible (Mellor and Gregory, 2003). Consciousness is suppressed *in utero* by a number of endogenous factors including allopregnanolone, pregnanolone, hypoxia, adenosine, prostaglandin D2 and warmth (Mellor *et al.*, 2005). Key steps during birth that provoke wakefulness are oxygenation derived from breathing air, and the effect this has in reducing adenosine concentrations in the bloodstream. Exposure to cold, physical stimulation (such as that resulting from licking or rubbing) and reduction in blood supply through the umbilicus are also important in initiating breathing. Breathing leads to the increase in oxygenation that allows consciousness to occur (Mellor and Diesch, 2006).

It cannot be claimed with certainty that there are no periods of transient or episodic conscious awareness in the fetus *in utero*, but, based on the electroencephalogram, no distinct phase of EEG activity has yet been identified that demonstrates the presence of this or any other type of wakefulness. The electroencephalogram of the fetus alternates between two types of sleep state: rapid eye movement (REM) sleep and non-REM (NREM) sleep. The interface between these two states has been discounted as a period when awareness is likely to occur (Mellor *et al.*, 2005). Not all of those who interpret EEG data would express certainty that the data obtained from fetal sheep in the latter stages of pregnancy could never indicate awareness. It would be widely accepted that the EEG evidence from the fetal brain supports the view that consciousness in the fetus is suppressed to some large degree before it breathes air. If there are episodes of conscious awareness in the fetus, they would probably coincide with periods of above-normal fetal oxygenation. Since (in the lamb fetus) the normal level of oxygenation is quite close to the level that is thought to be the interface between consciousness and unconsciousness in the neonatal lamb (Mellor and Gregory, 2003), it is possible that such episodes of consciousness could occur in the fetus. It has been suggested that consciousness is not an all-or-none phenomenon. Instead, there could be degrees of consciousness, and different depths of unconsciousness (Gregory and Shaw, 2000) often related to the disappearance of somatosensory reflexes.

For any species of animal, especially humans and domestic animals, we have information about the likelihood of a fetus surviving if removed from the uterus or egg. When this happens, the first question is: can the fetus start obtaining sufficient oxygen to be able to survive? For air-breathing animals, this means being able to breathe. Once they obtain oxygen, any suppression of consciousness is rapidly removed. Some animals can survive premature birth or hatching only if this is very shortly before the normal time of birth or hatching, while others can survive emergence when many weeks premature. Throughout the days or weeks when survival is possible, the young animal could become conscious if enough oxygen were obtained.

Reflex responses in the rat fetus are not necessarily signs of true pain experience. Appreciation of pain or distress requires functional maturation of higher brain centres, and it has been suggested that those centres are not sufficiently advanced in the near-term rat or human fetus to support those perceptions (Fitzgerald, 1999). Notwithstanding this, the fetus can show behavioural responses to relatively innocuous stimuli that resemble conscious responses. For example, intra-oral infusion of lemon juice elicits face-wiping behaviour in the rat fetus, whereas milk infusion evokes a stretch response similar to that seen post-natally (Robinson and Smotherman, 1992). The evidence that experience before birth or hatching can result in learning as well as responses indicates a degree of consciousness.

Circumstantial anecdotes considering whether or not human fetuses are conscious perinatally produce conflicting impressions. Some comments support the view that the human newborn is not conscious until it shows changes indicating that oxygenated blood is circulating after birth, whereas authors of other accounts consider that reflex responses *in utero* are indicative of awareness or an imprecise plane of conscious responsiveness.

9.3 Sentience in Young Individuals

It was thought until the 1970s that newborn human babies did not have a fully functional pain system, so operations involving cutting tissue were carried out without the use of anaesthetics or analgesics. A similar attitude existed in relation to young farm animals and pet animals. As explained above (Subsections 9.2.2 and 9.2.3), the pain system develops well before birth in mammals and there would be pain perception in young individuals unable to explain that they could feel pain.

When do developing humans reach the level of ability that a pig, dog, parrot or crow has? It is some years after birth before children can outperform these animals. For the first 1 or 2 years, human children cannot outperform some fish or cephalopods.

The development of the capabilities that are included as part of sentience is not inevitable in any given individual. The rearing conditions of animals have an effect on the stage at which they develop certain cognitive abilities. For example, for social species, confinement in conditions where normal social interaction is not possible affects the development of their behaviour. Broom and Leaver (1978) recorded abnormal behaviours in calves reared in individual pens that were not present if the animals were in groups of three. Individually housed calves show a variety of stereotypies, abnormalities of grooming and hair-eating behaviour, but also fail to show normal social interactions with the consequence that they adapted poorly when later put in a social group (de Paula Vieira *et al.*, 2012). Gaillard *et al.* (2014) found that calves kept in a social group were able to show reversal learning in a test where they had to move towards either a white or a red screen in order to obtain a reward. Isolation-reared calves, however, were not able to do this.

9.4 Sentience in Brain-damaged and Old Individuals

If the brain of an individual is damaged, the consequences can range from trivial to temporary loss of function to permanent prevention of all normal responses. Both the effects of traumatic injury to people and the effects of various kinds of dementia are described in many medical and a few veterinary publications. Only the general consequences of such conditions will be considered here. A further relevant research area is the effect of various methods for stunning animals, usually before slaughter.

The first category of individuals whose sentience will be considered here are those with brain damage, usually caused by trauma or a period with no blood supply to major brain areas, which prevents all normal function. These individuals can remain alive, sometimes controlling their own breathing and sometimes breathing only with assistance, but cannot respond to stimuli or control locomotor movements. Human patients with such a condition do not fulfil the criteria for sentience. A key question, however, is: what is the probability of a return to function that would constitute sentience? If there is no chance of such recovery, the individual is not and will not be sentient. If there is a potential for recovery, the individual would be considered sentient but temporarily not functioning.

A second category of individuals with brain malfunction are those whose injury or clinical brain disorder results in reduced cognitive function; this prevents the individual from having control over actions necessary for normal functioning and personal care and allows no prospect of recovery. There are many dementia patients in this category who cannot look after themselves but do still have some capacity to learn and remember, and to feel pain and fear. There is now evidence of links between brain changes and cognitive loss of various kinds (e.g. Cabeza *et al.*, 2005). The abilities of human patients with advancing dementia are often compared with those of young children. A patient might be unable to learn tasks that a child aged 2 to 4 years could learn. If compared with non-human animals, the abilities of many dementia patients would be substantially less than any of the animals that are considered sentient.

Many people with some brain malfunction, perhaps resulting from one of the forms of dementia, fluctuate in their abilities, being cognitively competent at some times and much less competent at other times. These individuals would be called sentient if they ever had the abilities commensurate with sentience. Those that lack some of the ability now but who are likely to recover it at some time in the future would also be called sentient.

Individuals may undergo periods of unconsciousness, during which they would not be aware or have pain or other feelings. People or other animals anaesthetized before an operation, and animals stunned before slaughter, would be in this category. All of these have the potential to return to a state where their sentience would be apparent so they continue to be sentient beings.

This will be obvious to most people, but perhaps it is also worthwhile to consider dead individuals. These are not sentient and do not have welfare. The dead will continue to affect the living via the memories of the living and any works, creations or other sources of influence that were produced during the lifetime of the individual.

9.5   Welfare During Development, After Brain Damage and During Old Age

Even though the mammalian fetus can show physical responses to external stimuli, some evidence suggests that full consciousness does not occur in the fetus until it starts to breathe air. However, it may be that the fluctuations in level of brain activity include periods when the fetus is conscious. It is known that events *in utero* can influence the behaviour of the individual once it is born, and some of those effects could be important to its subsequent welfare. The precocial species, which are well developed at birth, reach each level of functional development earlier, in terms of percentage of time *in utero* or *in ovo*, than altricial species. Precocial oviparous species present much evidence of being conscious at hatching and during the last days before hatching. If a mammal, bird or reptile is exposed to air before the normal birth or hatching time, it has the capacity for full consciousness by 50–60% of the developmental period. There is then the potential for a wide range of responses and for learning. The pain system can function after 50–80% of the developmental period.

Given the developmental facts, conclusions can be drawn about when sentience commences. For each kind of animal, we can determine when it could be conscious, perceiving and aware. During the latter period of development in a mammal, the individual may not be aware because some of its functions are suppressed in the absence of an availability of oxygen necessary for such functions. However, later in life we normally call an individual sentient when it is asleep or anaesthetized, because it has the potential to do all that a sentient being can do when awoken. The point during fetal development at which the individual is sentient should be considered to be that when there is the potential to be aware and to show the responses of a sentient being. This point may be after 50–70% of the developmental period up to birth or hatching, depending upon the species; perhaps 60% in humans. If procedures are carried out that might require anaesthesia or analgesia in a post-partum or post-hatching individual, then anaesthesia or analgesia should be used for the fetal individual.

We can consider and evaluate the welfare of any living animal, including one with severe brain damage. Even if a person would no longer be considered sentient because of brain damage, the extent to which coping mechanisms are functioning successfully can still be assessed. Good welfare in an unconscious person includes adequate breathing, temperature regulation, nutrition and water balance. The state of the individual when unconscious might be such that there would be negative effects after recovery of consciousness so the future welfare of the individual has to be considered. The same considerations obtain if the period of brain malfunction will be more than a few minutes or hours.

The welfare of any individuals is worse if they know that they are not coping adequately with the world in which they live. People in the early stages of dementia are often disturbed by their lack of ability to control things that they would have controlled when less affected by the dementia. The greater the perceived lack of control becomes, the worse the welfare will be. It may be possible to reassure people with dementia who have such concerns, but these are difficult problems and some poor welfare is still likely. Once the dementia sufferer has lost the ability to understand that they lack control over what is happening to them, their welfare may become better than it was when they were at the earlier stage of dementia progression.

Ethical Decisions About Humans and Non-humans

10

10.1 Ethical Decisions when Sentience has been Evaluated

As explained in Chapter 2, many decisions about which human actions are moral vary little across human societies, and have parallels in societies of other animals (Broom 2003, 2006c). Change has taken place, however, in what are considered to be the subjects of moral action. There is now concern about all people, not just those from the individual's own small community, and also about very young and very old humans and many kinds of animals. We are more likely to treat as deserving of moral consideration those identified as 'us' than those considered to be 'them'. At one time, categories of 'us' may well have included principally or only individuals readily recognized as close relatives. It is likely that the category expanded later to the wider range of individuals included if 'all of those who know who I am' is the category. Later, and still wider, is the group that 'might have access to the same information that I have', or 'all sentient beings who share characteristics with me'. Broom (2003) explains that for many people the latter three categories would include non-humans, and Midgley (1994) has pointed out that animals such as dogs have long been viewed as deserving moral consideration.

Many people want people and certain non-human animals to be protected solely because they are considered to have some intrinsic value (see discussion by Rollin, 1989). A further group of people, who may not hold such a view of intrinsic value, would say that apart from certain punishment situations it is wrong to cause people to suffer. Many of these people are also concerned that the welfare of animals should not be poor, again often with a statement that suffering should be prevented. When considering people, and with the 'intrinsic value' view, to cause the death of a person would always or usually be unacceptable. When considering other species, an animal's sudden and painless death would be a matter for great concern. However, with the view that welfare is the main concern, sudden and painless death would not be a concern. The position of many people is to have a strong view of the intrinsic value of people, some idea of the intrinsic value of other animals and a concern about the welfare of both humans and other animals. Some people, as Fraser (2008) points out, would consider that the prevention of poor welfare is something that has a preference value rather than a moral value. While it is mainly the moral value of individuals that is the issue considered here and by Broom (2010a), there are also aesthetic components of the values ascribed to people and other animals. Sometimes those perceived to be beautiful are valued more than those perceived to be ugly.

In deciding whether or not the killing of a human embryo is justified, whether or not a brain-damaged or senile person should be allowed to die, which animals should be killed for human use, and for which animals we have concern about welfare, many people take account of the cognitive and emotional functioning of the individual. The question of the sentience of the individual is important in such decisions. The words 'sentient beings' are used in some important legal documents, for example the Treaty of Amsterdam that is the basis for the EU as it now functions. The statement in this Treaty is 'Desiring to ensure improved protection and respect for the welfare of animals as sentient beings, have agreed . . .' (European Union, 1997: p. 110).

10.2   Summary of Which Animals are Sentient and When

How similar is the physiological and other functioning of humans and other animals? Much evidence has been presented in this book for similarities, and this is one of the reasons why a variety of animals are used as models for humans, for example in testing the toxicity of drugs and others substances to which humans are exposed. However, there are various differences in the enzymes that are present in animal species. As a consequence a substance that is useful and preferred in a species with the enzymes to use it may be toxic in another. For example, humans like chocolate but it is toxic to dogs. A comparison of toxicity in dogs and humans shows that, while they sometimes have the same metabolic pathways, dogs are often not good models for humans (Bailey *et al.*, 2013).

A prejudice exists to the effect that small animals are less likely to be sentient than large animals. However, it is not generally the case that the smaller members of any particular taxonomic group of animals have less behavioural complexity or cognitive ability than the larger members. When comparing across animal groups, hummingbirds and mice seem to live at a much faster pace than larger, slower-moving animals such as humans. Much decision making, often involving sophisticated brain processing, has to occur faster in such small animals than in large ones. When standing and watching hummingbirds feeding from a patch of flowers, I have sometimes been suddenly approached by one of them which hovered in front of me, looking at me for less than a second and then flew off extremely rapidly to resume feeding or take part in a social interaction. The human might well be perceived to be too slow to be of any consequence in a busy life. One measurement of ability that supports the idea that smaller animals can have better abilities than larger ones is the perception of temporal information (Healy *et al.*, 2013). When a measurement is made of the lowest frequency at which visual flicker is perceived, it is found that smaller animals perceive independent stimuli when larger animals perceive continuous images. Hence the smaller animals have better time resolution than larger animals. The fastest processing reported by Healy *et al.* was that of a blowfly, perhaps not a surprise to all who have tried to catch one. Perhaps blowflies perceive humans as slow and inconsequential.

As explained by Broom (2006d, 2007a) there are many ways in which the welfare of sentient animals can be poor. Actually or potentially harmful events might be more readily recognized and receive more attention as a result of the cognitive ability of the animal. For some sentient animals, pain can be especially disturbing on some occasions, because the individual concerned uses its sophisticated brain to appreciate that such pain indicates a major risk. However, more sophisticated brain processing will also provide better opportunities for coping with some problems. For example, humans may have means of dealing with pain that fish do not, and may suffer less from pain because they are able to rationalize that it will not last for long. Therefore, in some circumstances, humans who experience a particular pain might suffer more than fish, while in other circumstances a certain degree of pain may cause worse welfare in fish than in humans (Broom 2001b, 2006d). These arguments will also be valid for other causes of poor welfare. Fear is likely to be much greater in its impact if the context and risk cannot be analysed. In addition, more complex brains should allow more possibilities for pleasure, and this contributes greatly to good welfare. Accurate use of direct measures of animal welfare is the best way in which to decide how to treat individuals.

The evidence for cognitive awareness in fish is clear from a wide range of studies (Chapter 4, this volume; Bshary *et al.*, 2002; Chandroo *et al.*, 2004; Broom, 2007a). While we cannot know whether the feelings of fish are like our feelings, the criteria for sentience are fulfilled by at least those species of fish studied in this experimental work.

Experimental and observational studies of cognition and feelings in animals provide evidence that certain levels of ability and of functioning exist in some members of a species but they do not indicate that all members of the species are the same. There may be a substantial range in cognitive ability and emotional responsiveness within a species. However, if any member of a species is demonstrated to have significant cognitive ability, this should be taken into account when designing housing and husbandry systems for the species. Some of the ways in which cognitive ability can be considered when trying to improve the welfare of farm animals are discussed by Manteuffel *et al.* (2009).

Key issues in any discussion of the welfare of fish and invertebrates (Broom, 2007a) are: (i) whether they are aware of what is happening around them (Chandroo *et al.*, 2004); (ii) whether they are capable of cognitive processing; and (iii) whether they can have feelings such as pain (see Chapters 4–6). The general conclusion from the evidence presented on the functioning of fish, cephalopods and decapod crustaceans is that they are sentient. Information about cognition, pain and awareness in other invertebrate animals is presented in Chapter 4 and in Sections 4.2, 4.6, 5.5 and 6.4.

10.3   Animal Protection

The question to be considered here is: which animals should be protected? Should the range of protected animals be limited to warm-blooded animals, or vertebrate animals, or should it be extended to any of the invertebrate groups? Should protection begin at the point of hatching from an egg, or birth in the case of mammals, or should it begin at some point during fetal or embryonic development? At what point in development should there be protection? In practice, immature forms of which kinds of animals could be protected?

DeGrazia (1996: p. 69, pp. 226–231) considers sentience to be a condition for having interests and that there is no moral status without interests. For him, interests include preference interests that individuals have and which are associated with wants and desires, and welfare interests that are something which benefits the individual. Hence, DeGrazia argues (p. 93) that the capacity for responsiveness to stimuli is not sufficient for moral status and (p. 226) not all living beings have interests and hence moral significance.

Many people consider that sentience is a criterion for deciding which animals should be legally protected by laws, such as those concerning experimental animals in laboratories. Similarly, the use of anaesthetics and analgesics when serious sensitive tissue damage occurs may be decided according to whether or not the animal is sentient. The concept of welfare, however, applies to all animals so it is possible to assess the welfare of animals that are not sentient. Research on cognitive abilities of invertebrates has shown that those of cephalopods, decapod crustaceans, insects, spiders and some gastropod molluscs is greater than many biologists might have expected (Sherwin, 2001; Reznikova, 2003; Cross and Jackson, 2005; Broom, 2007a).

There is a general view among biologists and the public that there is a threshold level among animals above which protection should occur. Very few people would seek to protect protozoans or nematode worms but the vast majority would wish to protect primates, so a line based on scientific evidence has to be drawn somewhere between the two. If protection were limited to a group of animals that was too restricted, poor welfare could occur in animals used in experimental procedures. Risk assessment of this kind has to change according to the level of development of human knowledge. Our knowledge of the functioning of the brain and nervous system, and of animal welfare, has advanced rapidly in recent years. New knowledge has tended to show that the abilities and functioning of non-human animals are more complex than had previously been assumed. It is likely that future advances in knowledge will require reappraisal of the animals that should be protected.

The link between level of awareness and welfare is complex. Welfare concerns how well individuals are able to cope with good or bad environments (Broom and Johnson, 1993). Some animals, for example Protozoa, seem not to have any awareness and would not be called sentient. The welfare of sentient animals could be poor for more reasons than that of non-sentient animals because of the greater complexity of brain function of sentient animals. We should be concerned about the welfare of all animals but most people would be more concerned about those that are sentient. However, within this category of sentient animals, more sophisticated brain processing will provide better opportunities for coping with some problems. Humans seem to have means of dealing with pain that fish do not have. As a consequence, a certain degree of pain may cause worse welfare in fish than in humans (Broom, 2001b). This argument would also be valid for other causes of poor welfare. It also seems likely that more complex brains allow more possibilities for pleasure, which contributes greatly to good welfare. The same type of human action may sometimes be more cruel if inflicted on a simpler animal than on a human or other more complex animal.

Some practical questions about animal protection do not take account of sentience at all. A person may decide that a human should never be kept in captivity or killed for human benefit. The reasonable person deciding this may, however, allow exceptions where the human is a violent criminal, a soldier in a war, or a fetus at an early stage of development, so the qualities of the individual human are taken into account. The prohibition might be extended to a particular species of non-human animal. As soon as this position is adopted, there is a question about which animal species should be protected. That decision might be taken on the basis of sentience alone: for instance, no sentient animal should ever be kept in captivity or killed for human benefit. This would prevent the use of sentient animals as pets, or for transporting people, entertainment, food, clothing or medical research. In reality, very few people indeed would apply such rights-based arguments, either to humans or to other animals. In general, people have ethical positions on such subjects that take account of the welfare of the individual under consideration. Although there are decisions that are independent of welfare concerns, evaluation of effects on welfare is necessary for most decisions.

When the welfare of people and other animals is considered, the evaluation of welfare might be informed by knowledge of sentience, but is not dependent on it. As explained in several earlier chapters, welfare can be assessed without knowledge of the feelings of the individual or the potential for having feelings. Some animals do not have the capacity to have feelings. However, whenever the animal does have this capacity, the welfare assessment will take particular account of feelings as these are important biological mechanisms used to help individuals to cope with their environment. The major advantage of an understanding of the various component parts of sentience to an animal welfare scientist is to provide information on the likelihood of good or poor welfare in defined circumstances. For the general public, information about sentience informs decisions about which animal species should be protected in various ways.

An example of a practical decision for a person who uses an animal is whether or not anaesthesia and analgesia should be used if the treatment might be expected to cause pain. In many cases, the treatment involves cutting sensitive tissue as part of veterinary treatment or mutilations such as docking tails, ears or claws; castration; spaying; de-horning; beak-trimming; or caesarean section. Most people's ethical decision would be that, for sentient animals, pain relief should be mandatory for all occasions when pain is caused by such operations.

10.4   Conclusions About Sentience Research and Which Animals to Protect

The following list of conclusions, modified after Broom (2010a) is about what should be done in relation to studies of sentience and the treatment of animals:

1. When investigating brain and behaviour in humans and other animals, academics should use precise scientific methodology when describing observations, experimenting, analysing results and writing about these, but should not be afraid to use concepts such as emotion, feeling, mood, pain, fear, happiness, aware, consciousness, stress, need and welfare in presenting results. No concept should be avoided because there might be those who would criticize the use of complex concepts on the grounds that there must be parsimony in all description. If the subject is complex, some of the concepts must be complex.
2. Each concept used in cognition, awareness and animal welfare research should be properly defined in scientific writing rather than just being referred to in descriptive but imprecise ways.
3. An ability in individuals of a species does not necessarily mean that all members of the species have the ability, but the level of complexity of functioning of the animal should be taken into account when designing housing and husbandry systems for the species. Careful studies of animal welfare are required for this.
4. High levels of cognitive ability may often help animals to cope with their environment; hence a given level of a problem, such as pain, may be less in

more complex animals than in simpler animals. There is a possibility that animals may have fear of possible future adversity. The relationships between negative feelings such as fear and pain, and the role of cognition in the coping abilities of the animal, should be investigated further and considered when evaluating the risk of poor welfare. Cognitive ability should also be considered when designing methods of enriching the environments of captive animals.

5. A substantial body of research on parrots, dogs, pigs, cattle and other farm animals and companion animals shows that they have some ability for recognition, cognition, risk assessment, cognitive awareness, assessment awareness, emotions and feelings, and hence that they are sentient. Research on laboratory and wild mammals and birds is providing similar evidence. In particular, studies of birds in the crow family provide evidence of high levels of cognitive ability and awareness.

6. The information about learning, awareness and capacity for pain and other feelings in amphibians, reptiles, fish, cephalopods and decapod crustaceans is also clear enough to justify arguments for their protection if they are used in experimentation, for food or for other purposes. Learning and awareness in stomatopod crustaceans is at least equivalent to that in decapod crustaceans.

7. Spiders have substantial cognitive ability and perhaps executive awareness, and some insects such as bees and ants have quite high cognitive ability and probably assessment awareness. There is clear evidence for aspects of a pain system in gastropod molluscs, such as snails, slugs and swimming sea slugs, but we cannot be sure that these animals feel pain, or that they do not feel pain. Because some aspects of the pain system exist in leeches and swimming sea slugs, these animals are used as models for human pain. Evidence for a pain system is significantly less for insects and spiders than it is for molluscs. Cognitive ability and awareness in gastropod molluscs has not been shown to be as great as in some spiders and insects. There is a case for some degree of protection for spiders, gastropods and insects. However, the case is not as strong as that for vertebrates, cephalopods and decapod crustaceans at present.

8. All animal life should be respected and studies of the welfare of even the simplest invertebrate animals should be taken into account when we interact with these animals. Even if we do not protect the animals by law, we should try to avoid cutting an earthworm in half, mutilating a snail or damaging the wing of an insect.

10.5   Protection of the Unborn Child and Other Young

Almost every sperm and every egg has the potential to become part of a zygote and then a functioning individual. Once sperm and egg have fused to make a zygote, the probability of becoming an individual is increased but is usually still very low. In some species, birth or hatching alive means a high probability of becoming an adult but in others the odds against are still thousands to one. At what point in the long journey from egg or sperm to adult should we start to allocate inherent value to the individual? This is a question in relation to humans and other species whose fates we may control. It is a matter for law and for personal ethical decision.

If all have inherent value, it can logically be argued that every human sperm and egg should be protected. More frequently, it is argued that the zygote is of value because it has the potential to become an individual. This is true, even if most will not, and leads to the position that it is not acceptable to carry out any action that would be likely to result in a zygote not surviving. With this view, the use of contraceptive pills would not be acceptable. Once the implanted zygote has started to develop, if inherent value exists when there is potential to become an individual, this will not change until birth. However, most people take other factors into account when deciding on inherent value.

In addition to considering the likelihood of survival of the average sperm, egg, embryo, fetus, young animal or adult, it is also possible to assess at what stage independent survival is possible (see Section 9.2). Human premature babies do not survive if 21 weeks old, need considerable care if 22–25 weeks old and have decreasing risks of adverse effects as 37 weeks is approached. For some people, the earliest of the dates is the latest time at which an abortion would be acceptable.

Do we take account of sentience when considering whether or not abortion is acceptable? During pregnancy the fetus has a potential, increasing with time, of becoming a sentient individual. This argument is correct for humans and other sentient animals. However, the point at which the developing human fetus has the capacity for having feelings and being aware is about 60% through pregnancy. This corresponds to the age at which survival is possible.

At a time when it was thought that young animals (including human newborns) could not feel pain, operations involving opening the body cavity, removing the foreskin of the penis of young boys, and farm operations such as castration were carried out without anaesthetic or analgesic. As late as 1985, a young human infant in the USA was subject to operations involving cutting holes in the neck and opening the chest cavity after immobilization with a curare compound but no anaesthetic or analgesic. The anaesthesiologist involved said it had never been demonstrated that infants feel pain (Lee, 2002). With current knowledge, the use of pain relief is now normal for most operations on humans, many operations on pet animals and laboratory animals, but for few operations on farm and working animals.

10.6 Protection of Brain-damaged and Senile Persons and Other Animals

The word 'euthanasia', which means 'good death', should be used solely to mean killing an individual for the benefit of that individual. If the benefit is for someone else, it should be called 'killing' or 'humane killing' but not 'euthanasia' (Broom, 2007b). Euthanasia in humans is not legal in most countries, in particular because of difficulties in formulating a law that would not allow the possibility that old people might be encouraged to agree to hasten their death. However, in public discussions about the subject it is often stated that the expectation of loss of sentience might be a reason why a person would request euthanasia for themselves.

When a companion animal is suffering, the owner may decide that it would be better for that animal to be dead than to continue suffering. It is assumed that the animal is sentient and would prefer not to suffer further.

Sustainability, Welfare Attitudes and Education

11.1 Sustainability

When decisions are made about whether a system for exploiting resources should be used, an important question is whether or not the system is sustainable (Aland and Madec, 2009). The fact that something is profitable and there is a demand for the product is not now sufficient reason for the continuation of production. A system or procedure is sustainable if it is acceptable now and if its expected future effects are acceptable, in particular in relation to resource availability, consequences of functioning and morality of action (Broom, 2001c, 2014). A system might not be sustainable for several possible reasons. For animal usage systems, examples of such reasons are: (i) because it involves so much depletion of a resource that this will become unavailable to the system; (ii) because a product of the system accumulates to a degree that prevents the functioning of the system; or (iii) because members of the public find an action involved in it unacceptable. Where there is depletion of a resource or accumulation of a product, the level at which this is unacceptable, and hence the point at which the system is unsustainable, is usually considerably lower than that at which the production system itself fails. Other reasons for unacceptability are exemplified below. A system could be unsustainable because of harms to the perpetrator, other people, the environment, or other animals.

No system or procedure is sustainable if a substantial proportion of the local or world public now find aspects of it unacceptable, or if they consider now that its expected consequences in the future are morally unacceptable. Examples of unsustainable practices are discussed by Broom (2012). Adverse effects on people or animals can be reported in the media around the world and there are now consequences around the world of unacceptable practices in manufacturing, animal production or other human activities because of increased efficiency of communication.

Media reports of activities or events that the public find unacceptable may result in consumers in many countries refusing to buy animal and other products from the companies or countries involved: for example, dolphins caught in tuna nets, calves kept in small crates and sheep dying on an Australian ship going to Saudi Arabia (Broom, 2012).

11.2   Changing Ideas About Product Quality

The idea of quality for the goods that people buy has changed in the last 10–20 years. Quality referred formerly to immediately observable aspects: for an animal food product, its visual qualities and taste. These aspects of quality are still important, and expectations about taste are tending to become more refined, but other factors are now becoming incorporated into what constitutes good quality. Consumption has consequences and a higher proportion of these are now considered. If a food causes people to become sick, the quality is considered poor. If the food tends to make one fat, for some people the quality is considered poor. If food has added nutrients, some consider the quality to be better. In addition, a major recent change is that the ethics of the production method are taken into account. Factors considered by purchasers include: (i) the welfare of the animals used in production; (ii) any impact on the environment, including conservation of wildlife; (iii) ensuring a fair payment for producers, especially in poor countries; (iv) the preservation of rural communities so that the people there do not go to live in towns; and (v) the carbon footprint of each product, as factors leading to global warming are now high on the agenda of many discriminating consumers. The French 'Label Rouge' scheme led the way in this (Ouedraogo and Le Neindre, 1999) and the proportion of French consumers who bought only on price was already thought to have dropped to 25% by that time.

11.3   Attitudes to Animal Welfare and Consumer Pressure

Members of the public in all parts of the world, particularly in developed countries, are now insisting on transparency in commercial and governmental activities and on changes in methods of producing various products. There is a gradual changeover from a 'push society', driven in the case of animal production by the producers of the animals, to a 'pull society', driven by consumers and facilitated by governments and food retail companies

(Broom, 2010b, 2012). Increasing numbers of consumers now demand ethical production systems and refuse to buy products where production involves, for example, inhumane slaughter methods, rearing calves in small crates, unnecessarily killing dolphins in tuna nets, or the payment of very low prices to poor farmers in developing countries. As a consequence, many systems developed with consideration of only short-term market factors, even if widely used at present, are not sustainable. This means that, in some countries, the public has already demanded that such systems do not continue. Throughout the world, the public is likely to make such demands in the relatively near future. The first steps may be to set up supply for niche markets, but the rapidity of increase in consumer pressure is likely to lead to change away from the most unacceptable systems (Pollan, 2006). Changes with small economic cost are likely to occur faster than changes with more substantial cost. One of the first examples of consumers forcing change is the gradual disappearance, in increasing numbers of countries, of animal production procedures with poor welfare for the animals. A second example is the development of fair-trade systems and labelling schemes, which may eventually replace non-fair-trade products in supermarkets and other retail outlets. A possible future example may be that consumers will cease to tolerate very low biodiversity in farmed areas and buy only those products that can be produced from systems with moderate or high biodiversity.

Consumers drive legislation and retail company codes of practice for animal production (Bennett, 1994; Bennett *et al.*, 2002). Legislation on animal welfare has developed in the EU and in many countries because of pressure from voters (Broom, 2002, 2009). In general, the standards of retail companies have a substantially greater effect on the welfare of farm animals than legislation. The codes of practice of food companies have international impact. For example, many pig producers in Brazil have to comply with the animal welfare standards of UK supermarkets in order to sell to them; and egg producers in Thailand have to rear their birds according to the standards of the increasing numbers of US food chain companies that have animal welfare standards.

If food is not safe (if it contains damaging levels of toxins or pathogens) most consumers will never buy it however cheap it is. Individual food production companies are expected to be responsible for this aspect of food quality, but the public expects its government to ensure that adequate standards and adequate checking systems exist. The discovery of dioxin-contaminated animal feed and human food in Belgium (Bernard *et al.*, 2002) is an example of this. Incidents of this kind can have wide-ranging repercussions for governments, and companies can go bankrupt because the public becomes aware of such failures. There have always been concerns for animals and empathy with them. However, the extent of concern about animals in general has grown during the last 100–200 years (see Chapter 2). Consumers will refrain from purchasing animal products if they judge that the production procedures are unsustainable and thus not of good quality. Poor welfare of animals that are used in the production system is a major reason why some animal production systems are regarded by the public as unacceptable (Ryan, 1997). Hence these systems become unsustainable unless there is some modification to them. Animal welfare is becoming more important to members of the public as a reason for demanding change from farmers, food retail companies and governments. Members of the European Parliament receive more letters about animal welfare than about any other subject (Broom, 1999b). However, most people think about animal welfare issues infrequently, unless their attention is drawn to it by media coverage. When the information is brought to public attention, it appears that there is a level of animal welfare that is so poor that the majority of the public consider the system to be unacceptable. Hence animal welfare and public attitudes towards it must be considered whenever the sustainability of an animal production system is evaluated. Efforts to use systems of animal production that are acceptable in relation to preservation of biodiversity, good animal welfare, minimal carbon footprint and other aspects of sustainability are being developed (Broom *et al.*, 2013). In order to produce laws or codes of practice, scientific evidence is needed.

11.4   Welfare of Wild Animals, Including Pests

The attitudes of people to wild animals are often quite different according to the human activity that they affect or the human usage to which they are put. Predators, which attack humans or their domestic animals, were long regarded as targets for extermination by any means. Animals thought of as pests, for any reason, have been viewed in the same way. Different individual animals of the same species may be thought of and treated in quite different ways: for example, a person might be willing to cause substantial pain to a wild rabbit in a winter wheat field but be much less willing to cause the same pain to a rabbit in a laboratory cage or a cage on a rabbit farm, and be appalled at the idea of causing such pain to a child's pet rabbit (Broom, 1989). Similarly, a hunter thinks of a feral cat and a pet cat quite differently (Serpell, 1989). However, it does not matter to the animal what its impact on man is. When the welfare of an animal is assessed, this is done in exactly the same way whatever its human usage. Human moral obligations to the animals with which they interact are to minimize any poor welfare that results from the interaction, irrespective of the usage of the animal.

The wild animals that are viewed with affection by many members of the public are viewed as resources by those who exploit them. As a consequence, many of the wild animal welfare issues that are discussed are about whether or not methods of killing are humane. This is so for animals killed for food, those killed for fur production, and those such as elephants, rhinoceroses, whales and seals, which are killed for a range of other products. In addition, there are animals killed mainly for human entertainment such as the foxes and deer that are hunted with dogs, birds that are shot and fish that are caught by anglers. Animals regarded as pests may be trapped, poisoned, shot, excluded physically from potential feeding or resting areas, scared away from such areas, or changed physiologically (for example, sterilized). All of these actions will have effects on the welfare of the animals (Broom, 1999a).

When invertebrate animals are considered, respect for individuals and concern about welfare are affected by whether or not the animal is perceived to be a food item, or to be used in another way, or likely to harm humans or their resources. For example, lobsters, squid, oysters (e.g. *Ostrea edulis*) and escargots (edible snails, *Helix pomatia*) are thought of as items of food rather than as individual beings whose welfare may be considered. Indeed, those who consume them are more likely to blind themselves to any consideration of welfare, just as they do with other food animals. Similarly, researchers studying crickets (e.g. *Gryllus*) or the swimming marine sea slug *Aplysia* think of them principally as subjects for study. Most people think of wasps (*Vespa* spp.) solely as a somewhat dangerous nuisance, while spiders that are harmless and beneficial to humans are often killed because people do not like to see them or are afraid of them. Indeed, a factor that affects people's judgements about how animals should be treated is the aesthetic question of whether or not they are perceived to be beautiful. A butterfly may be pleasing to look at for many people. Those who look closely at marine worms such as *Phyllodoce maculata*, at many tubeworms, at nudibranch molluscs in the sea, or at the head of a honeybee or spider, usually find them beautiful. This response may make it more likely that individuals and populations of the animals will be preserved. Ethical decisions about how an animal should be treated should not be dominated by any of these factors.

Whale welfare can be assessed using many of the measures that are used for other animals (Broom, 2013). Whales are sentient, good at learning and have a pain system. In relation to the whale hunt, studies of welfare should consider the effects of: (i) the disturbance resulting from the approach of humans in boats; (ii) chasing by boats; (iii) a harpoon entering tissue; (iv) pulling on the line attached to the harpoon; (v) tissue damage by an explosive harpoon; and (vi) procedures during capture of individuals after they have been pulled to the whaling ship.

Where the welfare of a wild animal is perceived to be poor because the killing method is not reliably humane, consumers can refuse to buy products and laws banning their sale can be passed. However, the World Trade Organization (WTO) does not list animal welfare concerns as grounds for restricting trade. The EU has passed legislation banning trade in seal products on animal welfare grounds. This was the result of public pressure over many years because many of the young seals killed for their fur, principally in Canada, were not killed in a humane way (Broom, in press). Hence the argument for the ban was on public morality grounds, and stated that the poor welfare of the seals was a moral issue for EU citizens. The EU produced hardly any sealskin products so this action was not to do with competition with Canada. The EU ban was challenged at the WTO by Canada and this challenge was supported by Norway. A WTO panel was constituted entitled 'Dispute DS400 European Communities – Measures Prohibiting the Importation and Marketing of Seal Products' and hearings occurred in Geneva during 2013 (World Trade Organization, 2013). At these hearings Namibia and Iceland spoke in support of Canada, and other countries including Russia (which has a ban similar to that of the EU on animal welfare grounds) and the USA (which has a ban on conservation grounds) spoke in favour of the EU position.

Seals are either killed by a sealer walking to the seal and clubbing it, or by a person on a moving boat shooting a seal on an ice floe that is often moving, or by shooting a seal in the water. Clubbing and shooting can wound the seal or make the animal temporarily unconscious. Injured seals often enter the water and may escape. Herding or chasing seals will cause fear and other forms of poor welfare. The major question is whether or not there is a humane, acceptable method of killing seals. The arguments presented at the WTO by the EU referred to the evidence that seals are sentient beings but the bulk of the scientific arguments were about seal welfare: they were not about whether or not it is acceptable to kill seals. According to generally accepted principles, for example EU legislation and American Veterinary Medical Association guidelines (referring to commercial slaughter, killing for disease control and killing by a veterinarian), humane killing implies that: (i) the treatment of the animals in the course of the killing procedure does not cause poor welfare; and, (ii) if there is stunning, the stunning procedure results in instantaneous insensibility or, if the agent causing insensibility or death is a gas or injectable substance, no poor welfare occurs before insensibility and then death. It may be that the gas or injectable substance is not detectable by the animal. Careful injection has small effects so the killing method is still considered humane.

During a commercial seal hunt, some seals will be killed humanely. However, even if all rules are obeyed, the welfare of a substantial proportion of seals will be very poor. It was argued by the EU that it is not possible to stun and kill seals in commercial conditions without poor welfare in many seals. A key question is how seal killing compares with abattoir killing. Hence it is relevant to compare the rates of miss-stuns and delays in commercial sealing and abattoirs. In a series of papers on the Canadian seal hunt, the frequency of inaccurate stun, involving the need to repeat the stunning method, was much higher than in abattoirs. If a repeat stun is required in an abattoir this occurs within 3 s but sealers often could not get to the animals quickly, so the mean delay was longer, and often much longer. In addition, the Canadian government figures for seals struck and lost are a mean of 5%. These seals are injured and may take many hours or days to die. This does not occur in abattoirs.

On 25 November 2013 the WTO panel found that the EU Seal Regime does not violate Article 2.2 of the Technical Barriers to Trade (TBT) Agreement, that it fulfils the objective of addressing EU public moral concerns on seal welfare and that the seal hunt could not be changed to solve the problem. Following an appeal, in a decision on 22 May 2014, the WTO upheld that decision but said that EU exceptions to the ban, especially that for indigenous peoples, were not valid. This means that all seal products should be treated the same and all seal killing should be humane. This is a very important result as it is the first time that a product ban on animal welfare grounds, as part of public morality, has been accepted by the WTO. The possibility is raised that other product bans on the same grounds might be accepted.

11.5   GM Animals: Welfare and Public Attitudes

Conventional breeding methods need not affect welfare but can change animals in such a way that they have more difficulty in coping or are more likely to fail to cope (Broom, 1995, 2008b). One example of such an effect is the sensory, neurological or orthopaedic defects found commonly in certain breeds of dog. Others are the effects of the genes promoting obesity in mice, double muscling linked to parturition problems in cattle, and many examples of selection promoting fast growth and large muscles in farm animals. Modern strains of pigs have relatively larger muscle blocks, more anaerobic fibres and smaller hearts than have the ancestral strains (Dämmrich, 1987). They are more likely to die or to become distressed during any vigorous activity, for example during transport. Modern broiler strains grow to a weight of 2–2.5 kg in 35 days as compared with the 12 weeks they took to reach this weight 30 years ago. Their muscles and guts grow very fast but their skeleton and cardiovascular system do not. Hence many of the birds have leg problems (such as tibial dyschondroplasia or femoral head necrosis) or cardiovascular malfunction (often giving rise to ascites). Genetic selection of dairy cows for high milk production has led to increased leg disorders, mastitis and reproductive disorders, all of which are major welfare problems (Oltenacu and Broom, 2010).

Those aspects of modern biotechnology that are having or are likely to have the greatest impact on animal welfare are the use of genetically modified animals (GM animals) and cloning by nuclear transfer. The term 'GM animals' is used here to refer to animals whose genetic material has been altered using a method that does not occur naturally, but which excludes chemical or physical mutagenesis.

The first GM animal, a mouse, was made in the early 1980s (Gordon *et al.*, 1980; Palmiter, 1986) and this technology has been successfully applied to most mammals, including cattle, pigs and sheep (Hammer *et al.*, 1985; Simons *et al.*, 1988), poultry (Love *et al.*, 1994) and fish (Devlin *et al.*, 2001). Cloned amphibians were produced by Gurdon and collaborators in the 1970s; see review by Gurdon and Byrne (2003).

Microinjection was the earliest method of making GM animals, and electroporation has also been used. Both of these lead to mosaics: that is, genetic variability in the cells of the animal. Sperm-mediated gene transfer (SMGT) is the injection of a transgene vector, often viral, for GM. Androgenesis, gynogenesis and embryonic cell nuclear transplantation (ECNT) are used for cloning. Somatic cell nuclear transfer (SCNT) is used for cloning or for GM.

The effects of biotechnology procedures on animal welfare might be: (i) to improve it; (ii) to have no effect on it; or (iii) to make it poorer. What does the public consider to be positive or negative about GM and cloning? Some of the issues raised by scientific studies and public comments are listed in Tables 11.1 and 11.2.

Examples of some of the effects of genetic modifications of animals are: to benefit the animals by conferring disease resistance (Behboodi *et al.*, 2005); to

Table 11.1. Possible negative effects of cloning and GM.

1	Welfare problems – effects of the procedure (e.g. SCNT can lead to placental or fetal abnormality)
2	Welfare problems – effects of the transgene (e.g. insertion of the human growth hormone gene into pigs has caused major growth abnormalities)
3	Genetic uniformity in the population produced could increase the risk of disease epidemics
4	Effects on the safety of transgenic animal products for human consumption
5	Effects on wild animal populations of transgenic animals, particularly fish, that escape from captivity
6	Ethical and societal issues (e.g. equity of access to products by consumers, freedom to make ethical consumption choices)

SCNT, Somatic cell nuclear transfer.

Table 11.2. Possible positive effects of cloning and GM.

1	Improved welfare for the transgenic animals (e.g. due to deliberately enhanced disease resistance)
2	Reduction in the number of animals required for breeding programmes (cloning allows the copying of individuals so fewer are needed)
3	GM change to enhance nutritional value of animal products
4	Decreased pollution if GM increases animal digestion ability
5	Reduced cost of food, increased production of food
6	Engineering of animals suited to arid or other harsh environments

help to treat human disease by producing a blood clotting factor in sheeps' milk, (Houdebine, 2005); to develop new products for other purposes (Niemann and Kues, 2003); and to increase efficiency of animal production (Wheeler, 2003). Some people would accept none of these while others might accept them all. Many people would accept some with qualifications and a major reason for rejection is that animal welfare may be poorer.

There are effects of cloning procedures on animal welfare. Cloned common carp and rainbow trout are more variable and some do not survive well. A proportion of the cloned fish offspring are haploid and non-viable, while diploid hatchlings appear to have normal survival.

Birds cannot be fully cloned at present but there has been primordial germ cell transplantation, involving some cloned cells, in domestic chicks. The hatching rate of these birds was reduced by about 60% and survival of hatched chicks to adulthood was reduced by 20%.

Bovine clones have a high level of mortality, particularly *in utero*, where only 27% of pregnancies survive to term. There is also increased mortality in early life and cloned cattle often show developmental problems such as the large offspring syndrome. Many of these problems are a result of epigenetic abnormalities. If the clones survive the juvenile period there are usually no further welfare problems.

Cloned pigs show some increased early mortality and in the few animals studied the life expectancy was reduced. When sheep clones were produced, only 42% of pregnancies were maintained and only 50% of live-born lambs survived to weaning. For goat clones, 31% of pregnancies were maintained but 80% of live-born kids survived to weaning. In general, mortality and welfare problems are too high with SCNT. While there have been some improvements as a result of recent work, these procedures are not likely to be acceptable to the public or commercially viable.

The following are effects of genetic modification procedures on animal welfare. Most GM work is part of biomedical research, with a small amount of work involving farm animals, but most of the examples given here are for farm animals:

1. The production of the DNA often involves no animal welfare considerations because the source is tissue culture, human cells or animals that are killed humanely. However, if embryos or tissues must be removed from living animals in order to obtain the DNA, effects on welfare must be considered.
2. The production of the embryo for the insertion of DNA involves procedures used in producing lines of GM animals that may have welfare consequences for the welfare of the donor animals. For example: (i) the donor female may be injected with hormones to produce large numbers of oocytes; (ii) in large animals, artificial insemination may be used, sometimes using laparoscopy or laparotomy, to fertilize the oocytes; and (iii) embryo collection may involve killing the female or procedures such as oviduct flushing during laparotomic surgery. Each of these practices may involve welfare problems.
3. During micro-injection of DNA into the embryo, there is evidence that micro-injection of the transgene itself can lead to increased fetal loss. Many embryos injected with DNA die. However, this occurs at an early stage of development so is not a significant welfare problem.
4. When there is production of GM offspring, the insertion of the DNA construct within the genome can cause disruption of genes at that site, or there may be effects of the inserted gene. These effects may be apparent at birth, or may only become apparent at a later point in the animal's development, or when it is put under some kind of stress or put into a particular type of environment. The survival of transgenic, cloned offspring after SCNT in cattle is similar to or better than that of non-GM cloned animals. However, in pigs survival is somewhat worse. Alternatives to SCNT can result in fewer problems.
5. When GM animals are fostered onto normal females, the welfare of the fostered pups may be poor. Also, normal pups of the foster dam may have been killed to allow fostering of GM pups and the method of killing could affect welfare.
6. The consequence of the genetic change for the GM animals is a major animal welfare issue for laboratory animals because many of the GM animals are produced in order that they will be susceptible to developing pathological

conditions. For example, GM mice are produced that are likely to develop a tumour in order that anti-cancer treatments can be tested on them. Most people would say either that this should never be done, or that the tumour development should never be allowed to reach the point where the animal would suffer. Some genetic modifications lead to an unexpected malfunction. It is clearly necessary to use good-quality animal welfare science measures to check each GM line that might be continued in order that they will not be continued if such unwanted problems exist. No problems were revealed in a study of the behaviour of sheep genetically modified to produce human alpha-l-antitrypsin (used for treatment of human emphysema) in their milk (Hughes et al., 1996). However, the sheep did not live long. Salmon and other fish transgenic for a growth hormone gene have been produced. Many of these have an enlarged head and a bulging operculum. The problems become worse with increasing age.

Other positive and negative examples of genetic change effects include:

- GM catfish with a gene for cecropin are more resistant to enteric septicaemia.
- GM grass carp transgenic for human lactoferrin are resistant to haemorrhagic virus and Aeromonas hydrophila infection.
- Transgenic chickens that can synthesize RNA which interferes with influenza virus replication and packaging are less likely to suffer from or transmit the disease (Lyall et al., 2011). Some other GM chickens had positive and negative anti-disease consequences.
- Pigs transgenic for human growth hormone have many negative effects.
- Huber et al. (2012) assessed the welfare of a large number of pigs transgenic for the green fluorescent protein gene and found no deleterious effects.

An alternative to transgenesis is the direct administration of transgenes to the tissues of adult animals, resulting in a transient transgene expression in these tissues. Han et al. (2007) infused a vector carrying the bovine lactoferrin gene into the mammary glands of goats via the teat canal. Lactoferrin was expressed in the milk for up to about 1 week, with the potential to protect against mastitis. As in most GM studies, the consequences have not been evaluated using a range of welfare indicators.

The production of GM or cloned animals is allowed only in specified circumstances by the law in the UK and several other countries. The creation or duplication of favourite pets, or of animals intended as toys or as fashion accessories, would not be permitted. Table 11.3 summarizes the views of government committees, such as the UK Animal Procedures Committee and the public in the EU, about what is not acceptable in GM animal production.

While the majority of this section refers to genetic modification and cloning of animals, it is also necessary to consider carefully any proposed use of GM materials that would change an animal in some way. An example is the injection of a form of the hormone bovine somatotrophin (BST) produced

Table 11.3. What are publicly unacceptable consequences of genetic modification?

1	Animals should not be produced if they would be subject to harms of a degree and kind that ought under no circumstances to be inflicted upon an animal. This includes GM animals that would suffer severe or lasting distress, including animals to be created as disease models, unless there is clear evidence that the problems could be handled humanely
2	The production of GM animals should not occur if such work is likely to strip animals of their biological integrity, or render them incurably insentient
3	There should not be production of chimaeras, especially human–animal chimaeras, or of hybrids that involve a significant degree of hybridization between animals of very dissimilar kinds

by GM bacteria. Although BST is a naturally occurring hormone, the GM form is slightly different chemically and the amounts that can be given to the cows to increase milk production are much greater than that which would normally be present in the animals. The question considered by two EU scientific committees was whether or not there was scientific information about the consequences of the use of BST in the USA that would allow a decision about permission for its use in the EU. One report concerned animal welfare, the other human consumer health.

An assessment of the risk to consumers if dairy cows are regularly injected with recombinant BST was conducted (European Union Scientific Committee on Public Health, 1999). This identified a very small increased risk to consumers because of the effects on tumours of insulin-like growth factor 1 (IGF1) in milk. However, a much bigger effect on animal welfare was found. There was an increase in risk of clinical mastitis above the risk in non-treated cows, as demonstrated using meta-analyses or large data sets, of about 35%. BST increased the incidence of foot disorders 2.2 times with 2.1 times more days affected. The pregnancy rate dropped from 82% to 73% in multiparous cows and from 90% to 63% in primiparous cows, and multiple births were substantially increased. There were severe reactions at the injection site in at least 4% of cows. As a result of this information in a report (European Union Scientific Committee on Animal Health and Animal Welfare, 1999), the use of BST was banned in the EU and in many other countries.

Conclusions as a result of such information are that:

1. Moral issues associated with biotechnology will be considered by the public and should be taken into account at an early stage in any biotechnology research.
2. One of the possible consequences of the use of GM products or GM animals is on animal welfare. Many different systems for coping with the environment should be considered when assessing welfare. These systems interact and health is an important part of welfare in such assessments.

3. A checklist for animal welfare should be further developed for general cage-side use in the case of GM animals.

4. When sold, every GM product for use with animals and every GM animal should have details of properly tested effects on animal welfare.

11.6   Welfare Legislation

Legislation has effects on how people house and manage animals. As explained above, it is generally initiated by pressure from voters on elected politicians. In a scientific area the politicians need to know the latest state of scientific knowledge on the subject. As a consequence, the EU has set up scientific committees on a range of subjects. Previous committees considering animal welfare were the Scientific Veterinary Committee, Animal Welfare Section and the Scientific Committee on Animal Health and Animal Welfare. The present committee is the European Food Safety Authority (EFSA) Scientific Panel on Animal Health and Welfare. This has a parallel with the Food and Drug Administration (FDA) in the USA. A difference from the FDA is: (i) that many aspects of sustainability, including animal welfare, are part of the work of EFSA; and (ii) that the reports and opinions produced by EFSA are by committees of independent scientists, appointed solely on the grounds of their scientific expertize. They are not representatives of countries or interest groups and all scientists have to declare any interest that could possibly affect their evidence. In producing scientific reports, all statements have to be supported by information that is published and refereed. A significant part of their work is the assessment of risks and benefits (Broom, 2006d).

The subject area covered by EFSA is wide, reflecting the public concern. The reports of the panel that deals with animal disease and animal welfare have led to changes in EU legislation and scientifically based standards in Europe and elsewhere in the world. A scientific committee producing reports on animal welfare is of value in any major country. Measures to check that there is compliance with legislation exist in the Member States of the EU and in other countries.

Legislation within European countries and EU Directives and Regulations have usually been preceded by Recommendations from Council of Europe committees such as the Standing Committee of the European Convention on the Protection of Animals Kept for Farming Purposes. This committee produced recommendations including those on poultry kept for egg production, pigs, cattle, animals used for fur production, sheep, goats, chickens kept for meat production and ducks. There are other Conventions on the protection of pet animals, animals for slaughter, animals used for experimentation and animals during transport. The information in the Conventions and Recommendations has formed the basis for legislation and codes of practice in many countries.

On a worldwide scale the Organisation Internationale des Epizooties (World Organisation for Animal Health, OIE) is now producing sets of recommendations that are likely to be treated as if they were laws by most nations in the world, just as OIE recommendations on animal disease are respected.

What do we need from animal welfare law? Most people would say that the law should prevent people from causing poor welfare in animals, including pain, fear, other suffering, severe disease, distress caused by environments which do not meet the animals' needs, or distress caused by the genetic selection used in breeding. In reality, the way that a law might do this is principally by acting as a deterrent. People who disobey the law are punished and this becomes known. Whether it is explicit or implicit in a law, there will be a principle that guides the actions of those aware of the law. Laws should provide guidance, not just a mechanism to punish (Radford, 2001). One key point of the UK Animal Welfare Law is that it refers directly to animal welfare. A second is that it refers to people having a duty of care to the animals covered by the law. The effectiveness of laws and codes depends on the attitudes of people to them and on the efficacy of enforcement.

In order that the ethics of the production method can be taken into account properly, products must be traceable. If foods can be traced, it is less likely that toxins, other poor-quality materials or pathogens will be in them. If animals can be traced, the sources of animal disease outbreaks are more likely to be found and places where injuries, or other causes of poor welfare, occurred are more likely to be found (Broom, 2006e). Legislation and industry initiatives ensuring traceability are important.

Current EU legislation on animal welfare deals with the keeping of various farm animal species, the transport of animals, stunning and killing of animals, laboratory procedures and other matters intended to prevent poor welfare in domestic and some wild animals. Since animal health is such an important part of animal welfare, all legislation that prevents or minimizes animal disease has major benefits for animal welfare. The legislation on the training of veterinarians and that prohibiting the trapping of animals or the killing of wild animals, whether formulated principally for conservation or welfare reasons, is also important in relation to animal welfare.

The sequence of events that lead to a Directive or Regulation about animal use in the EU always includes the production of a scientific report by unbiased scientists. As an example of events leading to an EU Directive, the welfare of calves may be considered (Broom, 2009). From 1960 onwards there was some public concern that close confinement and inadequate diet lead to poor welfare in calves reared for veal production. This was a focus of the book *Animal Machines* by Harrison (1964) that led to the setting up of a national committee on farm animal welfare in the UK. In the 1970s and 1980s research results gave evidence of serious welfare problems in closely confined calves. In 1988 the recommendation concerning the welfare of cattle from the Council of Europe Standing Committee on the Protection of Animals Kept for Farming Purposes stated that cattle should be able to make all normal movements for such behaviours as grooming and exercise. Some European countries passed legislation banning calf crates. The 1990 report by a group of scientists coordinated by the European Commission was followed in 1991 by Directive 91/629/EEC laying down minimum standards for the protection of calves. This Directive allowed calves to be kept in crates that did not allow them to turn around, specifying a minimum width, but also required a report on calf welfare in relation to housing and management from the EU Scientific Veterinary Committee by 1 October 1997 so that Ministers could reconsider the Directive. In the 1990s there was further welfare research on such things as the effects of diet, confinement and space in groups on calf welfare, and in 1994–1995 there was much public pressure for action. An early scientific report was requested so in 1995 the 'Report on the welfare of calves' was produced by the EU Scientific Veterinary Committee, Animal Welfare Section. In 1996 there was a proposal for legislation from European Commission staff and the scientific report was considered by Ministry staff from each Member State. A revised proposal was discussed by Ministers from each Member State and the 1997 Directive 97/2/EC phasing out the use of veal crates and inadequate diets was passed.

Similarly, within the EU, the Council Regulation (EC) 1/2005 'On the protection of animals during transport and related operations' takes up some of the recommendations of two separate reports: (i) the EU Scientific Committee on Animal Health and Animal Welfare Report 'The welfare of animals during transport (Details for Horses, Pigs, Sheep and Cattle)' (March, 2002); and (ii) the European Food Safety Authority 'Report on the welfare of animals during transport' (2004) which deals with the other species. There are now many other examples of legislation based on information from scientific reports in the EU and elsewhere.

Those who formulate laws, such as government ministers or the staff of the European Commission, have to take account of all factors in determining the best course of action so they are never just risk managers (see Section 8.7). Much of what they are trying to achieve is benefit, not just reduction of risk. This is true in legislation to reduce disease and to promote good health as well as, more obviously, in the animal welfare area. Legislation can promote good welfare and it often does (Broom, 2014).

The actual effect of legislation on the welfare of animals depends upon the responses of those owning and managing the animals. This response, in turn, depends upon the nature of any enforcement. Some systems for farm animal production will not continue if they are made illegal because they depend upon large manufacturers who are easily forced to change to a legal system. Other aspects of legislation can be enforced only by checks including those on farms, transport vehicles, markets and slaughterhouses, and the extent of law-breaking will be significantly affected by the frequency and quality of the checks. For many transgressions, unannounced inspections are necessary if transgressors are to be discovered. There are regional and national differences in the seriousness with which legislation is viewed by those involved in the animal production business.

11.7 Welfare and Codes of Practice

Farmers often sell animals or their products such as milk or eggs to single purchasers who represent large retail chains or wholesale distribution companies. The increase in direct selling to supermarket chains has led to considerable power being placed in the hands of these companies. It is possible for these purchasers to lay down conditions for animal production and to enforce these by inspection. The standards set by the supermarket chains are determined by what people will buy and by their reputation with the public.

The public image of large companies that retail food, including supermarket chains and fast-food companies, is of great importance to them. Bad publicity because of a risk to public health, a risk to the environment or the occurrence of poor welfare at any stage of the production process, can be very damaging. Hence it is in the interest of such food companies to avoid any scandal that might threaten their good image. When these companies receive many letters from consumers complaining about a product that they sell, they have to take notice of the points being made.

As a consequence of consumer pressure, food retail companies are adopting standards that they impose on their suppliers. In some cases, these standards are quite simple: for example, the supermarket chain Albert Hein in the Netherlands and elsewhere limited its sales of eggs to 'scharreleie', which meant that the hens were reared in conditions where they could scratch in litter. Marks & Spencer in the UK and elsewhere stopped selling eggs from battery cages. In other cases, elaborate standards have been described in detail and sent to suppliers. One of the first systematic attempts to provide comprehensive information about the conditions under which animals were kept in the course of food production was the 'Freedom Foods' scheme run by the Royal Society for the Prevention of Cruelty to Animals (RSPCA) in the UK. In this scheme, the standards for housing and management have been set by a widely respected animal protection society and farms are inspected by Freedom Foods staff. Retailers who subscribe to the scheme are allowed to use the Freedom Foods logo, which is accepted as honest by the purchasing public. Acceptance by the public of products which are produced in such a way that the welfare of the animals is good depends upon trust in the organization carrying out the labelling and inspection. Some large supermarket chains and other food retailers are trusted because it is thought that they could not afford to be found out if they were not labelling and policing adequately.

The enforcement of standards by food retailers has led to substantial changes in the welfare of animals on farms because every producer has to conform to the standards in order to sell its products. The rapid development of such schemes in several countries has, in general, been based on scientific evidence about animal welfare.

11.8   Education: Animal Abilities and Welfare

11.8.1   Teaching animal welfare: non-university courses

Objective information about animal welfare is now widely available on the internet as well as in books and papers. A particularly useful source of information is Animal Welfare Science Hub (http://animalwelfarehub.com, also available at www.animal-welfare-indicators.net/site/index.php/global-hub). Such sites are run by animal welfare scientists so are not biased. There is also useful information at the sites of several universities, at animal protection societies such as the World Society for the Protection of Animals (WSPA, www.wspa-international.org/wspaswork/education/concepts-animal-welfare-modules.aspx) and at the Food and Agriculture Organization (FAO, www.fao.org/ag/againfo/themes/animal-welfare/aw-abthegat/aw-whaistgate/en).

Some aspects of animal welfare teaching can be made available for the primary and secondary school level, for animal producers, animal handlers, transport drivers, slaughterhouse staff, laboratory technicians, veterinary inspectors and others (Gallo *et al.*, 2010).

11.8.2   Teaching animal welfare: university courses

There has been rapid refinement of concepts in animal welfare science and development of a wide range of sophisticated measurements of welfare. The education of veterinary, animal science and biology students has not kept pace with these developments, so there is an urgent need for animal welfare courses to be designed and taught in universities. Professionals such as veterinarians also need Continuing Veterinary Education courses in animal welfare.

Animal welfare should be taught to veterinary and animal science students in a separate course because: (i) the scientific subject is interdisciplinary so integrated lectures are needed; (ii) the students need guidance on the inter-relations of the ethics and the science, for example to understand deontological and utilitarian approaches; and (iii) it is necessary to separate scientific evaluation from ethical judgement because animal welfare is not an evaluative discipline.

What is the best sequence for animal welfare courses? Most well-structured university courses on animal welfare include the following (Hewson *et al.*, 2005; Broom, 2005, 2010b):

1. An early introduction to some of the problems (Year 1, first term).
2. Basic science courses including: sensory, adrenal, brain function, behaviour, immune system function, pathology, animal husbandry systems, the concept of sentience.
3. Animal welfare course including:
  • concepts;
  • ethics;

- scientific assessment (the wide range of physiological, behavioural and other measures of welfare, including pain, fear and other positive and negative feelings, in a wide range of animals, wild and domestic;
- integration of measures, long-/short-term, magnitude of good or poor welfare;
- species housing, handling, transport, disease, mutilations, slaughter topics;
- effects of genetic selection, human contact; and
- possibilities for practical monitoring on-farm or otherwise *in situ.*

4. Legal and social aspects, animal welfare in relation to sustainability and ideas of product quality.

References

Abbott, N.J., Williamson, R. and Maddock, L. (eds) (1995) *Cephalopod Neurobiology – Neuroscience Studies in Squid, Octopus, and Cuttlefish*. Oxford University Press, Oxford, UK.

Agrillo, C., Dadda, M., Serena, G. and Bisazza, A. (2009) Use of number by fish. *PLOS ONE* 4, e4786.

Aland, A. and Madec, F. (eds) (2009) *Sustainable Animal Production*. Wageningen Academic Publishers, Wageningen, Netherlands.

Alexander, R.D. (1979) *Darwinism and Human Affairs*. University of Washington Press, Pullman, Washington.

Allen, C. and Bekoff, M. (2007) Animal consciousness. In: Schneider, S. and Velmans, M. (eds) *Blackwell Companion to Consciousness*. Blackwell, London, pp. 58–71.

Altemus, M., Redwine, I.S., Leong, Y.-M., Frye, C.A., Porges, S.W. and Carter, C.S. (2001) Responses to laboratory psychosocial stress in postpartum women. *Psychosomatic Medicine* 63, 814–821.

Anand, K.J.S. and Hickey, P.R. (1987) Pain and its effects in the human neonate and foetus. *New England Journal of Medicine* 317, 1321–1329.

Anderson, J.R., Kuroshima, H., Paukner, A. and Fujita, K. (2009) Capuchin monkeys (*Cebus apella*) respond to video images of themselves. *Animal Cognition* 12, 55–62.

Arey, D.S. (1992) Straw and food as reinforcers for prepartal sows. *Applied Animal Behaviour Science* 33, 217–226.

Arey, D.S. (1997) Behavioural observations of peri-parturient sows and the development of alternative farrowing accommodation: a review. *Animal Welfare* 6, 217–229.

Aristotle (330 BC) Rhetoric, Book 2, Chapter 1, 1378a.

Bahnick, L., Moss, L. and Fadil, C. (1996) Development of visual self-recognition in infancy. *Ecological Psychology* 8, 189–208.

Bailey, J., Thew, M. and Balls, M. (2013) An analysis of the use of dogs in predicting human toxicology and drug safety. *ATLA* 41, 335–350.

Baldock, N.M. and Sibly, R.M. (1990) Effects of handling and transportation on heart rate and behaviour in sheep. *Applied Animal Behaviour Science* 28, 15–39.

Balm, P.H.M. and Pottinger, T.G. (1995) Corticotrope and melanotrope POMC-derived peptides in relation to inter-renal function during stress in rainbow trout (*Oncorhynchus mykiss*). *General Comparative Endocrinology* 98, 279–288.

Barr, S., Laming, P., Dick, J.T.A. and Elwood, R.W. (2008) Nociception or pain in a decapod crustacean? *Animal Behaviour* 75, 745–751.

Barton, R.A. and Dunbar, R.I.M. (1997) Evolution of the social brain. In: Whiten, A. and Byrne, R.W. (eds) *Machiavellian Intelligence II*. Cambridge University Press, Cambridge, UK, pp. 240–263.

Bates, L.A. and Byrne, R.W. (2007) Creative or created: using anecdotes to investigate animal cognition. *Methods* 42, 12–21.

Bateson, P. (1991) Assessment of pain in animals. *Animal Behaviour* 42, 827–839.

Behboodi, E., Ayres, S.L., Memili, E., O'Coin, M., Chen, L.H., Reggio, B.C., Landry, A.M. *et al.* (2005) Health and reproductive profiles of malaria antigen-producing transgenic goats derived by somatic cell nuclear transfer. *Cloning Stem Cells* 7, 107–118.

Beilharz, R.G. (1985) Special phenomena. In: Fraser, A.F. (ed.) *World Animal Science A5. Ethology of Farm Animals*. Elsevier, Amsterdam, Netherlands, pp. 363–370.

Bekoff, M. and Sherman, P.W. (2004) Reflections on animal selves. *Trends in Ecology and Evolution* 19, 176–180.

Bennett, R.M. (1994) (ed.) *Valuing Farm Animal Welfare*. University of Reading, Reading, UK.

Bennett, R.M., Anderson, J. and Blaney, R.J.P. (2002) Moral intensity and willingness to pay concerning farm animal welfare issues and the implications for agricultural policy. *Journal of Agricultural and Environmental Ethics* 15, 187–202.

Bentham, J. (1789) *An Introduction to the Principles of Morals and Legislation*. T. Payne, London.

Bergamo, P., Maldonado, H. and Miralto, A. (1992) Opiate effect on the threat display in the crab *Carcinus mediterraneus*. *Pharmacology Biochemistry and Behavior* 42, 323–326.

Bernard, A., Broeckaert, F., De Poorter, G., De Cock, A., Hermans, C., Saegerman, C. and Houins, G. (2002) The Belgian PCB/dioxin incident: analysis of the food chain contamination and health risk evaluation. *Environmental Research* 88, 1–18.

Berridge, K.C. (1996) Food reward: brain substrates of wanting and liking. *Neuroscience and Biobehavioral Reviews* 20, 1–25.

Bertenthal, B. and Fisher, K. (1987) Development of self-recognition in the infant. *Developmental Psychology* 14, 44–50.

Berthe, F., Vannier, P., Have, P., Serratosa, J., Bastino, E., Broom, D.M., Hartung, J. and Sharp, J.M. (2012) The role of EFSA in assessing and promoting animal health and welfare. *EFSA Journal* 10(10), s1002, 19–27.

Beukema, J.J. (1970) Angling experiments with carp decreased catchability through one trial learning. *Netherlands Journal of Zoology* 20, 81–92.

Block, N. (1991) Evidence against epiphenomenalism. *Behavioral Brain Science* 14, 670–672.

Block, N. (1998) How can we find the neural correlate of consciousness? *Trends in Neuroscience* 19, 456–459.

Blokhuis, H.J., Veissier I., Miele, M. and Jones, B. (2010) The Welfare Quality project and beyond: safeguarding farm animal well-being. *Acta Agriculturae Scandinavica, Section A, Animal Science* 60, 129–140.

Blood, D.C. and Studdert, V.P. (eds) (1988) *Baillière's Comprehensive Veterinary Dictionary*. Baillière Tindall, London.

Boal, G.J., Hylton, R.A., Gonzalez, S.A. and Hanlon, R.T. (1999) Effects of crowding on the social behavior of cuttlefish (*Sepia officinalis*). *Contemporary Topics in Laboratory Animal Science* 38, 49–55.

Boissy, A., Manteuffel, G., Jensen, M.B., Moe, R.O., Spruijt, B., Keeling, L.J., Winckler, C. *et al.* (2007) Assessment of positive emotions in animals to improve their welfare. *Physiology and Behavior* 92, 375–397.

Bokkers, E.A.M., Vries, M. de, Antonissen, I.C.M.A. and Boer, I.J.M. de (2012) Inter- and intra-observer reliability of experienced and inexperienced observers for the Qualitative Behaviour Assessment in dairy cattle. *Animal Welfare* 21, 307–318.

Bonadonna, F. and Sanz Aguilar, A. (2012) Kin recognition and inbreeding avoidance in wild birds: the first evidence for individual kin-related odour recognition. *Animal Behaviour* 84, 509–513.

Box, H.O. and Gibson, K.R. (eds) (1999) *Mammalian Social Learning: Comparative and Ecological Perspectives. Symposia of the Zoological Society of London* 72. Cambridge University Press, Cambridge, UK.

Boyle, P.R. (1987) *Cephalopod Life Cycles*, Vol 2. Academic Press, London.

Bradshaw, R.H. (1998) Consciousness in non-human animals: adopting the precautionary principle. *Journal of Consciousness Studies* 5, 108–114.

Braithwaite, V.A. and Huntingford, F.A. (2004) Fish and welfare: do fish have the capacity for pain perception and suffering. *Animal Welfare* 13, 587–592.

Brambell, F.W.R. (1965) *Report of the Technical Committee to Enquire into the Welfare of Animals Kept Under Intensive Husbandry Conditions*. HMSO, London.

Brantas, G.C. (1980) The pre-laying behaviour of laying hens in cages with and without laying nests. In: Moss, R. (ed.) *The Laying Hen and its Environment. Current Topics in Veterinary Medicine Animal Science* 8. Martinus Nijhoff, The Hague, pp. 227–234.

Broad, K.D., Mimmack, M.I., Keverne, E.B. and Kendrick, K.M. (2002) Increased BDNF and trk-B mRNA expression in cortical and limbic regions following formation of a social recognition memory. *Journal of Neuroscience* 16, 2166–2174.

Broglio, C., Rodriguez, F. and Salas, C. (2003) Spatial cognition and its neural basis in teleost fishes. *Fish and Fisheries* 4, 247–255.

Brookshire, K.H. and Hoegnander, O.C. (1968) Conditioned fear in the fish. *Psychological Reports* 22, 75–81.

Broom, D.M. (1981a) *Biology of Behaviour*. Reprinted 2009. Cambridge University Press, Cambridge, UK.

Broom, D.M. (1981b) Behavioural plasticity in developing animals. In: Garrod, D.R. and Feldman, J.D. (eds) *Development in the Nervous System. British Society for Developmental Biology Symposium* 5. Cambridge University Press, Cambridge, UK, pp. 361–378.

Broom, D.M. (1983) The stress concept and ways of assessing the effects of stress in farm animals. *Applied Animal Ethology* 11, 79.

Broom, D.M. (1986) Indicators of poor welfare. *British Veterinary Journal* 142, 524–526.

Broom, D.M. (1987) Applications of neurobiological studies to farm animal welfare. In: Wiepkema, P.R. and van Adrichem, P.W.M. (eds) *Biology of Stress in Farm Animals: An Integrated Approach. Current Topics in Veterinary Medicine and Animal Science* 42. Martinus Nijhoff, Dordrecht, Netherlands, pp. 101–110.

Broom, D.M. (1988) The scientific assessment of animal welfare. *Applied Animal Behaviour Science* 20, 5–19.

Broom, D.M. (1989) Ethical dilemmas in animal usage. In: Paterson, D. and Palmer, M. (eds) *The Status of Animals*. CAB International, Wallingford, UK, pp. 80–86.

Broom, D.M. (1991a) Animal welfare: concepts and measurement. *Journal of Animal Science* 69, 4167–4175.

Broom, D.M. (1991b) Assessing welfare and suffering. *Behavioural Processes* 25, 117–123.

Broom, D.M. (1994) The valuation of animal welfare in human society. In: Bennett, R.M. (ed.) *Valuing Farm Animal Welfare*. University of Reading, Reading, UK, pp. 1–7.

Broom, D.M. (1995) Measuring the effects of management methods, systems, high production efficiency and biotechnology on farm animal welfare. In: Mepham, T.B., Tucker, G.A. and Wiseman, J. (eds) *Issues in Agricultural Bioethics*. Nottingham University Press, Nottingham, UK, pp. 319–334.

Broom, D.M. (1998) Welfare, stress and the evolution of feelings. *Advances in the Study of Behavior* 27, 371–403.

Broom, D.M. (1999a) The welfare of vertebrate pests in relation to their management. In: Cowan, P.D. and Feare, C.J. (eds) *Advances in Vertebrate Pest Management*. Filander Verlag, Fürth, Germany, pp. 309–329.

Broom, D.M. (1999b) Welfare and how it is affected by regulation. In: Kunisch, M. and Ekkel, H. (eds) *Regulation of Animal Production in Europe*. KTBL, Darmstadt, Germany, pp. 51–57.

Broom, D.M. (2000) Welfare assessment and problem areas during handling and transport. In: Grandin, T. (ed.) *Livestock Handling and Transport*, 2nd edn. CAB International, Wallingford, UK, pp. 43–61.

Broom, D.M. (2001a) The use of the concept animal welfare in European conventions, regulations and directives. In: *Food Chain*. Conference proceedings, Uppsala. SLU Services, Uppsala, Sweden, pp.148–151.

Broom, D.M. (2001b) Evolution of pain. In: Soulsby, E.J.L. and Morton, D. (eds) *Pain: Its Nature and Management in Man and Animals. Royal Society of Medicine International Congress and Symposium Series* 246, 17–25.

Broom, D.M. (2001c) Coping, stress and welfare. In: Broom, D.M. (ed.) *Coping with Challenge: Welfare in Animals including Humans*. Dahlem University Press, Berlin, pp. 1–9.

Broom, D.M. (2002) Does present legislation help animal welfare? *Landbauforschung Völkenrode* 227, 63–69.

Broom, D.M. (2003) *The Evolution of Morality and Religion*. Cambridge University Press, Cambridge, UK, pp. 259.

Broom, D.M. (2005) Animal welfare education: development and prospects. *Journal of Veterinary Medical Education* 32, 438–441.

Broom, D.M. (2006a) Adaptation. *Berliner und Münchener Tierärztliche Wochenschrift* 119, 1–6.

Broom, D.M. (2006b) Behaviour and welfare in relation to pathology. *Applied Animal Behaviour Science* 97, 71–83.

Broom, D.M. (2006c) The evolution of morality. *Applied Animal Behaviour Science* 100, 20–28.

Broom, D.M. (2006d) Introduction – Concepts of animal protection and welfare including obligations and rights. In: *Animal Welfare. Ethical Eye Series*. Council of Europe Publishing, Strasbourg, France, pp. 13–28.

Broom, D.M. (2006e) Traceability of food and animals in relation to animal welfare. In: *Annals of the 2nd International Conference on Agricultural Product Traceability*. Ministry of Agriculture, Livestock and Food Supply, Brasilia, pp. 195–201.

Broom, D.M. (2007a) Cognitive ability and sentience: which aquatic animals should be protected? *Diseases in Aquatic Organisms* 75, 99–108.

Broom, D.M. (2007b) Quality of life means welfare: how is it related to other concepts and assessed? *Animal Welfare* 16 (Suppl.), 45–53.

Broom, D.M. (2008a) Welfare assessment and relevant ethical decisions: key concepts. *Annual Review of Biomedical Sciences* 10, T79–T90.

Broom, D.M. (2008b) Consequences of biological engineering for resource allocation and welfare. In: Rauw, W.M. (ed.) *Resource Allocation Theory Applied to Farm Animal Production.* CAB International, Wallingford, UK, pp. 261–274.

Broom, D.M. (2009) Animal welfare and legislation. In: Smulders, F. and Algers, B.O. (eds) *Welfare of Production Animals: Assessment and Management of Risks.* Wageningen Pers., Wageningen, Netherlands, pp. 341–354.

Broom, D.M. (2010a) Cognitive ability and awareness in domestic animals and decisions about obligations to animals. *Applied Animal Behaviour Science* 126, 1–11.

Broom, D.M. (2010b) Animal welfare: an aspect of care, sustainability, and food quality required by the public. *Journal of Veterinary Medical Education* 37, 83–88.

Broom, D.M. (2011) A history of animal welfare science. *Acta Biotheoretica* 59, 121–137.

Broom, D.M. (2012) Defining agricultural animal welfare: from a sustainability and product quality viewpoint. In: Pond, W.E., Bazer, F.W. and Rollin, B.E. (eds) *Animal Welfare in Animal Agriculture.* CRC Press, Boca Raton, Florida, pp. 84–91.

Broom, D.M. (2013) The welfare of invertebrate animals such as insects, spiders, snails and worms. In: Kemp, T.A. van der and Lachance, M. (eds) *Animal Suffering: From Science to Law. International Symposium.* Éditions Yvon Blais, Paris, pp. 135–152.

Broom, D.M. (in press) International perspectives on animal welfare science and policy. In: Cao, D. and White, S. (eds) *Animal Law.* Springer, Berlin.

Broom, D.M. and Fraser, A.F. (2007) *Domestic Animal Behaviour and Welfare,* 4th edn. CAB International, Wallingford, UK.

Broom, D.M. and Johnson, K.G. (1993) *Stress and Animal Welfare,* Reprinted with corrections 2000. Kluwer, Dordrecht, Netherlands.

Broom, D.M. and Leaver, J.D. (1978) The effects of group-rearing or partial isolation on later social behaviour of calves. *Animal Behaviour* 26, 1255–1263.

Broom, D.M. and Zanella, A.J. (2004) Brain measures which tell us about animal welfare. *Animal Welfare* 13, S41–S45.

Broom, D.M., Sena, H. and Moynihan, K.L. (2009) Pigs learn what a mirror image represents and use it to obtain information. *Animal Behaviour* 78, 1037–1041.

Broom, D.M., Galindo, F.A. and Murgueitio, E. (2013) Sustainable, efficient livestock production with high biodiversity and good welfare for animals. *Proceedings of the Royal Society B* 280 (1771), 2013–2025.

Brown, D.E. (1991) *Human Universals.* Temple University Press, Philadelphia, Pennsylvania.

Bshary, R., Wickler, W. and Fricke, H. (2002) Fish cognition, a primate's eye view. *Animal Cognition* 5, 1–13.

Budelmann, B.U. (1998) Autophagy in octopus. *South African Journal of Marine Science* 20, 101–108.

Burghardt, G.M. (1985) Animal awareness. *American Psychologist* 40, 905–919.

Burghardt, G.M. (2009) Ethics and animal consciousness: how rubber the ethical ruler? *Journal of Social Issues* 65, 499–521.

Burman, O.H.P., Parker, R.M.A., Paul, E.S. and Mendl, M. (2008) A spatial judgement task to determine background emotional state in laboratory rats *Rattus norvegicus. Animal Behaviour* 76, 801–809.

Burt de Perera, T. (2004) Fish can encode order in their spatial map. *Proceedings of the Royal Society, London B* 271, 2131–2134.

Butler, A.B. and Hodos, W. (2005) *Comparative Vertebrate Neuroanatomy, Evolution and Adaptation.* Wiley, New York.

Byrne, R. (1995) *The Thinking Ape: Evolutionary Origins of Intelligence.* Oxford University Press, Oxford, UK.

Byrne, R.W. (1997) Machiavellian intelligence. *Evolution and Anthropology* 5, 172–180.

Byrne, R.W. and Bates, L.A. (2007) Sociality, evolution and cognition. *Current Biology* 17, R714–R723.

Byrne, R.W. and Bates, L.A. (2010) Primate social cognition: uniquely primate, uniquely social or just unique? *Neuron* 65, 815–830.

Cabanac, M. (1979) Sensory pleasure. *Quarterly Review of Biology* 54, 1–29.

Cabanac, M. (1992) Pleasure: the common currency. *Journal of Theoretical Biology* 155, 173–200.

Cabeza, R., Nyberg, L. and Park, D. (eds) (2005) *Cognitive Neuroscience of Aging: Linking Cognitive and Cerebral Aging.* Oxford University Press, Oxford, UK.

Caldwell, R.L. (1986) The deceptive use of reputation by stomatopods. In: Mitchell, R.W. and Thompson, N.S. (eds) *Deception.* SUNY Press, Albany, New York, pp. 129–145.

Call, J. and Carpenter, M. (2001) Do apes and children know what they have seen? *Animal Cognition* 4, 201–220.

Carew, T.J. and Sahley, C.L. (1986) Invertebrate learning and memory: from behavior to molecules. *Annual Review of Neuroscience* 9, 435–487.

Carey, M.P. and Fry, J.P. (1993) A behavioural and pharmacological evaluation of the discriminative stimulus induced by pentylenetetrazole in the pig. *Psychopharmacology* 111, 244–250.

Carey, M.P. and Fry, J.P. (1995) Evaluation of animal welfare by the self-expression of an anxiety state. *Laboratory Animals* 29, 370–379.

Carruthers, P. (2000) *Phenomenal Consciousness: A Naturalistic Theory.* Cambridge University Press, Cambridge, UK.

Carter, C.S. (2001) Is there a neurobiology of good welfare? In: Broom, D.M. (ed.) *Coping with Challenge: Welfare of Animals Including Human.* Dahlem University Press, Berlin, pp. 11–30.

Carter, C.S. and Altemus, M. (1997) Integrative functions of lactational hormones in social behaviour and stress management. *Annals of the New York Academy of Sciences* 807, 164–174.

Chandroo, K.P., Duncan, I.J.H. and Moccia, R.D. (2004) Can fish suffer? Perspectives on sentience, pain, fear and stress. *Applied Animal Behaviour Science* 86, 225–250.

Cheney, D.L. and Seyfarth, R.M. (1990) *How Monkeys See the World.* University of Chicago Press, Chicago, Illinois.

Clayton, N.S. and Dickinson, A. (1998) Episodic-like memory during cache-recovery by scrub jays. *Nature* 395, 272–274.

Clore, G.A. and Ortony, A. (2000) Cognition in emotion: always, sometimes or never? In: Lane, R.D. and Nadel, L. (eds) *Cognitive Neuroscience of Emotion.* Oxford University Press, Oxford, UK, pp. 24–61.

Concise Oxford English Dictionary (2011) *Concise Oxford English Dictionary.* Oxford University Press, Oxford, UK.

Coppinger, R. and Coppinger, L. (2001) *Dogs: A Startling New Understanding of Canine Origin, Behavior and Evolution.* Scribner, New York.

Council of Europe (1999) *Standing Committee of the European Convention for the Protection of Animals kept for Farming Purposes (T-AP) Recommendation concerning domestic ducks* (Anas platyrhynchos). Council of Europe, Strasbourg, France.

Cronin, G.M. and Wiepkema, P.R. (1984) An analysis of stereotyped behaviour in tethered sows. *Annales de Recherches Vétérinaires* 15, 263–270.

Crook, J. (1988) The experiential context of intellect. In: Byrne, R.W. and Whiten, A. (eds) *Machiavellian Intelligence: Social Expertise and the Evolution of Intellect in Monkeys.* Clarendon Press, Oxford, UK, pp. 347–362.

Cross, F.R. and Jackson, R.R. (2005) Spider heuristics. *Behavioural Processes* 69, 125–127.

Curtis, S.E. (1983) Perception of thermal comfort by farm animals. In: Baxter, S.H., Baxter, M.R. and MacCormack, J.A.C. (eds) *Farm Animal Housing and Welfare. Current Topics of Veterinary Medicine Animal Science* 24. Martinus Nijhoff, The Hague, pp. 59–66.

Czanyi, V. and Doka, A. (1993) Learning interactions between prey and predator fish. *Marine Behaviour and Physiology* 23, 63–78.

Damasio, A.R. (2000) *The Feeling of What Happens*. Vintage, London.

Damasio, A.R., Grabowski, T.J., Bechara, A., Damasio, H., Ponto, L.L., Parvisi, J. *et al.* (2000) Sub-cortical and cortical brain activity during the feeling of self-generated emotions. *Nature Neuroscience* 3, 1049–1056.

Dämmrich, K. (1987) Organ change and damage during stress – morphological diagnosis. In: Wiepkema, P.R. and van Adrichem, P.W.M. (eds) *Biology of Stress in Farm Animals: An Integrated Approach*. Martinus Nijhoff, Dordrecht, Netherlands, pp. 71–81.

Dantzer, R. (2002) Can farm animal welfare be understood without taking into account the issues of emotion and cognition? *Journal of Animal Science* 80, E1–E9.

Dantzer, R. and Mormède, P. (1979) *Le stress en Élevage Intensif*. Masson, Paris.

Dawkins, M. (1983) Battery hens name their price: consumer demand theory and the measurement of animal needs. *Animal Behaviour* 31, 1195–1205.

Dawkins, M. (1993) *Through Our Eyes Only*. Freeman, Oxford, UK.

Dawkins, M.S. (1980) *Animal Suffering: The Science of Animal Welfare*. Chapman and Hall, London.

Dawkins, M.S. (1990) From an animal's point of view: motivation, fitness and animal welfare. *Behavioral and Brain Sciences* 13, 1–31.

Dawkins, M.S. (2006) Through animal eyes: what animal behaviour tells us. *Applied Animal Behaviour Science* 100, 4–10.

Dawkins, M.S. (2012) *Why Animals Matter: Animal Consciousness, Animal Welfare and Human Well-being*. Oxford University Press, Oxford, UK.

Dawkins, R. (1976) *The Selfish Gene*. Oxford University Press, Oxford, UK.

DeGrazia, D. (1996) *Taking Animals Seriously*. Cambridge University Press, Cambridge, UK.

Dennett, D.C. (1984) *Elbow Room: The Varieties of Free Will Worth Wanting*. MIT Press, Cambridge, Massachusetts.

de Paula Vieira, A., de Passillé, A.-M. and Weary, D.M. (2012) Effects of the early social environment on behavioral responses of dairy calves to novel events. *Journal of Dairy Science* 95, 5149–5155.

Désiré, I, Boissy, A. and Veissier, I. (2002) Emotions in animals: a new approach to animal welfare in applied ethology. *Behavioural Processes* 60, 165–180.

Désiré, I., Veissier, I., Després, G. and Boissy, A. (2004) On the way to assess emotions in animals: do lambs evaluate an event through its suddenness, novelty or unpredictability? *Journal of Comparative Psychology* 118, 363–374.

Désiré, I., Veissier, I., Després, G., Delval, E., Toporenko, G. and Boissy, A. (2006) Appraisal process in sheep: interactive effect of suddenness and unfamiliarity on cardiac and behavioural responses. *Journal of Comparative Psychology* 120, 280–287.

Devlin, R.H., Biagi, C.A., Yesaki, T.Y., Smailus, D.E. and Byatt, J.C. (2001) Growth of domesticated transgenic fish. *Nature* 409, 781–782.

Dickinson, A. and Balleine, B. (2002) The role of learning in the operation of motivational systems. In: Poshler, H. and Gallistol, R. (eds) *Stevens Handbook of Experimental Psychology*. John Wiley, New York, pp. 497–533.

Doyle, R.E., Lee, C., Deiss, V., Fisher, A.D., Hinch, G.N. and Boissy, A. (2011) Measuring judgement bias and emotional reactivity in sheep following long-term exposure to unpredictable and aversive events. *Physiology and Behavior* 102, 503–510.

Dubner, R. (1994) Methods of assessing pain in animals. In: Wall, P.D. and Melzack, R. (eds) *Textbook of Pain*, 3rd edn. Churchill Livingstone, Edinburgh, pp. 293.

Dunbar, R.I.M. (2000) Causal reasoning, mental rehearsal and the evolution of primate cognition. In: Heyes, C. and Huber, L. (eds) *The Evolution of Cognition*. MIT Press, Cambridge, Massachusetts, pp. 205–219.

Duncan, I.J.H. (1978) The interpretation of preference tests in animal behaviour. *Applied Animal Ethology* 4, 197–200.

Duncan, I.J.H. (1992) Measuring preferences and the strength of preferences. *Poultry Science* 71, 658–663.

Duncan, I.J.H. (1993) Welfare is to do with what animals feel. *Journal of Agricultural and Environmental Ethics* 6 (Suppl. 2), 8–14.

Duncan, I.J.H. (2006) The changing concept of animal sentience. *Applied Animal Behaviour Science* 100, 11–19.

Duncan, I.J.H. and Petherick, J.C. (1991) The implications of cognitive processes for animal welfare. *Journal of Animal Science* 69, 5017–5022.

Duncan, I.J.H. and Wood-Gush, D.G.M. (1971) Frustration and aggression in the domestic fowl. *Animal Behaviour* 19, 500–504.

Duncan, I.J.H. and Wood-Gush, D.G.M. (1972) Thwarting of feeding behaviour in the domestic fowl. *Animal Behaviour* 20, 444–451.

Dwyer, C.M. and Lawrence, A.B. (2008) Introduction to animal welfare and the sheep. In: Dwyer, C.M. (ed.) *The Welfare of Sheep*. Springer, Berlin, pp. 1–40.

Dyakonova, V.E. (2001) Role of opioid peptides in behavior of invertebrates. *Journal of Evolutionary Biochemistry and Physiology* 37, 335–347.

EFSA (2005) Aspects of the biology and welfare of animals used for experimental and other scientific purposes (Report and Opinion). *EFSA Journal* 292, 1–136.

EFSA (2006a) The risks of poor welfare in intensive calf farming systems. *EFSA Journal* 366, 1–36.

EFSA (2006b) Animal health and welfare risks associated with the import of wild birds, other than poultry, into the European Union. *EFSA Journal* 410, 1–55.

EFSA (2009) Scientific report on the effects of farming systems on dairy cow welfare and disease. Also scientific opinions on the same subject. *EFSA Journal* 1143, 1–38.

EFSA (2012a) Statement on the use of animal-based measures to assess the welfare of animals. *The EFSA Journal* 10(6), 2767.

EFSA (2012b) Scientific opinion on the use of animal-based measures to assess welfare in pigs. *The EFSA Journal* 10(1), 2512.

EFSA (2012c) Guidance on risk assessment for animal welfare. *The EFSA Journal* 10(1), 2513.

EFSA (2012d) Scientific opinion on the use of animal-based measures to assess welfare of dairy cows. *The EFSA Journal* 10(1), 2554.

EFSA (2012e) Scientific opinion on the use of animal-based measures to assess welfare of broilers. *The EFSA Journal* 10(7), 2774.

Ehrensing, R.H., Michell, G.F. and Kastin, A.J. (1982) Similar antagonism of morphine analgesia by MIF–1 and naloxone in *Carassius auratus*. *Pharmacology, Biochemistry and Behaviour* 17, 757–761.

Eich, E. and Macaulay, D. (2000) Fundamental factors in mood-dependent memory. In: Forgas, J.P. (ed.) *Feeling and Thinking: The Role of Affect in Social Cognition*. Cambridge University Press, Cambridge, UK, pp. 109–130.

Eisner, T. (1993) In defense of invertebrates. *Experientia* 49, 1.

Elliker, K. (2007) Social cognition and its implications for the welfare of sheep. PhD thesis, University of Cambridge, Cambridge, UK.

Elwood, R.W. (2012) Evidence for pain in decapod crustaceans. *Animal Welfare* 21 (S2), 23–27.

Elwood, R.W. (2013) Can we infer pain in crustaceans from behaviour experiments? In: Kemp, T.A. van der and Lachance, M. (eds) *Animal Suffering: From Science to Law*. International Symposium. Éditions Yvon Blais, Paris.

Elwood, R.W. and Appel, M. (2009) Pain experience in hermit crabs. *Animal Behaviour* 77, 1243–1246.

Elwood, R.W., Barr, S. and Patterson, L. (2009) Pain and stress in crustaceans. *Applied Animal Behaviour Science* 118, 128–136.

Emery, N.J. and Clayton, N.S. (2001) Effects of experience and social context on prospective caching strategies by scrub jays. *Nature* 414, 443–446.

Engel, J.R. and Engel, J.G. (1990) *Ethics of Environment and Development: Global Challenge and International Response*. Belhaven Press, London.

European Union (1997) Treaty of Amsterdam amending the Treaty on European Union, the treaties establishing the European Communities and certain related acts (97/C 340/01). http://eur-lex.europa.eu/legal-content/EN/TXT/PDF/?uri=CELEX:11997D/TXT&qid=1404130806690&from=EN (accessed 30 June 2014).

European Union (2007) European Union Treaty of Lisbon. http://europa.eu/lisbon_treaty/full_text/index_en.htm (accessed 13 March 2014).

European Union Scientific Committee on Animal Health and Animal Welfare (1999) Report on animal welfare aspects of the use of bovine somatotrophin. ec.europa.eu/food/fs/sc/scah/out21_en.pdf (accessed 24 March 2014).

European Union Scientific Committee on Public Health (1999) Report on public health aspects of the use of bovine somatotrophin. ec.europa.eu/food/fs/sc/scv/out19_en.html (accessed 24 March 2014).

Favre, J.-Y. (1975) *Comportement d'Ovins Gardés*. Ministère de l'Agriculture Ecole Nationale Superieure Agronomique de Montpelier, Monpelier, France.

Feld, M., Dimant, B., Delorenzi, A., Coso, O. and Romano, A. (2005) Phosphorylation of extra-nuclear ERK/MAPK is required for long-term memory consolidation in the crab *Chasmagnathus*. *Behavioural Brain Research* 158, 251–261.

Fiorito, G. (1986) Is there 'pain' in invertebrates? *Behavioural Processes* 12, 383–388.

Fitzgerald, M. (1999) Development and neurobiology of pain. In: Wall, P.D. and Melzack, R.D. (eds) *Textbook of Pain*, 4th edn. Churchill Livingstone, Edinburgh, pp. 235–251.

Flecknell, P. (2001) Recognition and assessment of pain in animals. In: Soulsby, Lord and Morton, D. (eds) *Pain: Its Nature and Management in Man and Animals*. International Congress and Symposium Series 246, 63–68.

Forgas, J.P. (ed.) (2000) *Handbook of Affect and Social Cognition*. Lawrence Erlbaum Associates, Mahwah, New Jersey.

Forkman, B.A. (2002) Learning and cognition. In: Jensen, P. (ed.) *The Ethology of Domestic Animals*. CAB International, Wallingford, UK, pp. 51–64.

Fox, E. (2008) *Emotion Science*. Palgrave Macmillan, Basingstoke, UK.

Fraser, D. (1999) Animal ethics and animal welfare science: bridging the two cultures. *Applied Animal Behaviour Science* 65, 171–189.

Fraser, D. (2008) *Understanding Animal Welfare: The Science in its Cultural Context.* Wiley Blackwell, Chichester, UK.

Fraser, D. and Matthews, L.R. (1997) Preference and motivation testing. In: Appleby, M.C. and Hughes, B.O. (eds) *Animal Welfare.* CAB International, Wallingford, UK, pp. 159–171.

Fraser, D., Weary, D.M., Pajor, E.A. and Milligan, B.N. (1997) The scientific conception of animal welfare that reflects ethical concerns. *Animal Welfare* 6, 187–205.

Fraser, D., Duncan, I.J.H., Edwards, S.A., Grandin, T., Gregory, N.G., Guyonnet, V., Hemsworth, P.H. *et al.* (2013) General principles for the welfare of animals in production systems: the underlying science and its application. *The Veterinary Journal* 198, 19–27.

Gaillard, C., Meagher, R.K., Keyserlink, M.A.G. von and Weary, D.M. (2014) Social housing improves dairy calves' performance in two cognitive tests. *PLOS ONE* 9(2), e90205.

Gallo, C., Tadich, N., Huertas, S., César, D., Paranhos da Costa, M. and Broom, D.M. (2010) Animal welfare education in Latin America. *Proceedings of the International Conference on Animal Welfare Education: Everyone is Responsible.* Brussels, 1–2 October 2010. European Union, DG SANCO, Brussels, pp. 90–97.

Gallup, G.G. (1982) Self-awareness and the emergence of mind in primates. *American Journal of Primatology* 2, 237–248.

Gallup, G.G. (1983) Towards a comparative psychology of mind. In: Mellgren, R.L. (ed.) *Animal Cognition and Behaviour.* North Holland Publishing, New York, pp. 502–503.

Gallup, G.G. (1998) Self-awareness and the evolution of social intelligence. *Behavioural Processes* 42, 239–247.

Gallup, G., Andersen, J.R. and Shillito, D.J. (2002) The mirror test. In: Bekoff, M., Allen, C. and Burghardt, G.M. (eds) *The Cognitive Animal: Empirical and Theoretical Perspectives on Animal Cognition.* MIT Press, Boston, Massachusetts, pp. 326–333.

Gert, B. (1988) *Morality: A New Justification of the Moral Rules.* Oxford University Press, New York.

Gherardi, F. and Atema, J. (2005) Memory of social partners in hermit crab dominance. *Ethology* 111, 271–285.

Giannakoulopoulos, X., Sepulveda, W., Kourtis, P., Glover, V. and Fisk, N.M. (1994) Fetal plasma cortisol and β-endorphin response to intra-uterine needling. *Lancet* 344, 77–81.

Goodall, J. (1963) Feeding behaviour of wild chimpanzees: a preliminary report. *Symposium of the Zoological Society of London* 10, 39–48.

Gordon, J.W., Scangos, G.A., Plotkin, D.J., Barbosa, J.A. and Ruddle, F.H. (1980) Genetic transformation of mouse embryos by microinjection of purified DNA. *Proceedings of the National Academy of Sciences USA* 77, 7380–7384.

Greenspan, R.J. and Swinderen, B. van (2004) Cognitive consonance: complex brain functions in the fruit fly and its relatives. *Trends in Neurosciences* 27, 707–711.

Gregory, N.G. (2004) *Physiology and Behaviour of Animal Suffering.* Blackwell, London.

Gregory, N.G. and Shaw, F.D. (2000) Penetrating captive bolt stunning and exsanguinations of cattle in abattoirs. *Journal of Applied Animal Welfare Science* 3, 215–230.

Griffin, D.R. (1984) *Animal Thinking.* Harvard University Press, Cambridge, Massachusetts.

Grind, W. van de (1997) *Natuurlijke Intelligentie.* Nieuwezijds, Amsterdam, Netherlands.

Grind, W. van de (2002) Physical, neural, and mental timing. *Consciousness and Cognition* 11, 241–264.

Gumert, M.D., Kluck, M. and Malaivijitnond, S. (2009) The physical characteristics and usage patterns of stone axe and pounding hammers used by long-tailed macaques in the Andaman Sea region of Thailand. *American Journal of Primatology* 71, 594–608.

Gurdon, J.B. and Byrne, J.A. (2003) The first half-century of nuclear transplantation. *Proceedings of the National Academy of Sciences USA* 100, 1048–1052.

Gygax, L., Reefmann, N., Wolf, W. and Langbein, J. (2013) Pre-frontal cortex activity, sympatho-vagal reaction and behaviour distinguish between situations of feed reward and frustration in dwarf goats. *Behavioural Brain Research* 239, 104–114.

Hagen, K. and Broom, D.M. (2003) Cattle discrimination between familiar herd members in a learning experiment. *Applied Animal Behaviour Science* 82, 13–28.

Hagen, K. and Broom, D.M. (2004) Emotional reactions to learning in cattle. *Applied Animal Behaviour Science* 85, 203–213.

Hammer, R.E., Pursel, V.G., Rexroad Jr, C.E., Wall, R.J., Bolt, D.J., Ebert, K.M., Palmiter, R.D. and Brinster, R.L. (1985) Production of transgenic rabbits, sheep and pigs by microinjection. *Nature, London* 315, 680–683.

Hampton, R.R. (2001) Rhesus monkeys know when they remember. *Proceedings of the National Academy of Sciences* 98, 5359–5362.

Han, Z.-S., Li, Q.-W., Zhang, Z.-Y., Xiao, B., Gao, D.-W., Wu, S.-Y., Li, J. *et al.* (2007) High-level expression of human lactoferrin in the milk of goats by using replication-defective adenoviral vectors. *Protein Expression and Purification* 53, 225–231.

Haney, J. and Lukowiak, K. (2001) Context learning and the effect of context on memory retrieval in *Lymnaea*. *Learning and Memory* 8, 35–43.

Hanlon, R.T. and Messenger, J.B. (1996) *Cephalopod Behaviour*. Cambridge University Press, Cambridge, UK.

Harcourt, A. (1992) Coalitions and alliances: are primates more complex than non-primates? In: Harcourt, A.H. and Waal, F.B.M. de (eds) *Coalitions and Alliances in Primates and Other Animals*. Oxford University Press, Oxford, UK, pp. 445–471.

Harding, E.J., Paul, E.S. and Mendl, M. (2004) Cognitive bias and affective state. *Nature* 427, 312.

Harrison, R. (1964) *Animal Machines*. Vincent Stuart, London; reprinted with commentaries by CAB International, Wallingford, UK, 2013.

Harwood, D. (1928) *Love for Animals and How It Developed in Great Britain*. Columbia University Press, New York. Republished 2002 as Preece, R. and Fraser, D. (eds) *Dix Harwood's Love for Animals and How It Developed in Great Britain*. Edwin Mellen Press, Lewiston, New York.

Hauber, M.E. and Sherman, P.W. (2001) Self-referant phenotype matching: theoretical considerations and phenotype matching. *Trends in Neuroscience* 24, 609–616.

Hauser, M. (2000) *Wild Minds: What Animals Really Think*. Henry Holt, New York.

Haynes, R.P. (2008) Animal and human health and welfare. A comparative philosophical analysis. *Journal of Agricultural and Environmental Ethics* 21, 91–97.

Healy, K., McNally, L., Ruxton, G.D., Cooper, N. and Jackson, A.L. (2013) Metabolic rate and body size are linked with perception of temporal information. *Animal Behaviour* 86, 685–696.

Heijningen, C.A.A. van, Chen, J., van Laatum, I., van der Hulst, B. and ten Cate, C. (2013) Rule learning by zebra finches in an artificial grammar learning task: which rule? *Animal Cognition* 16, 165–175.

Held, S. and Spinka, M. (2011) Animal play and animal welfare. *Animal Behaviour* 81, 891–899.

Held, S., Mendl, M., Devereux, C. and Byrne, R.W. (2000) Social tactics of pigs in a competitive foraging task: the 'informed forager' paradigm. *Animal Behaviour* 59, 569–576.

Held, S., Mendl, M., Laughlin, K. and Byrne, R.W. (2002) Cognition studies with pigs: livestock cognition and its implications for production. *Journal of Animal Science* 80, E10–E17.

Helton, W.S. (2005) Animal expertise, conscious or not. *Animal Cognition* 8, 67–74.

Hemmer, H. (1983) *Domestikation: Verarmung der Merkwelt*. Vieweg, Braunschweig, Germany.

Hemsworth, P.H. and Coleman, G.J. (1998) *Human–Livestock Interaction: The Stockperson and the Productivity and Welfare of Intensively Farmed Animals*. CAB International, Wallingford, UK.

Hewson, C.J., Baranyiova, E., Broom, D.M., Cockram, M.S., Galindo, F.A., Hanlon, A.J., Hanninen, L. *et al.* (2005) Approaches to teaching animal welfare at 13 veterinary schools world wide. *Journal of Veterinary Medical Education* 32, 422–437.

Heyes, C. (2000) Evolutionary psychology in the round. In: Heyes, C. and Huber, L. (eds) *The Evolution of Cognition*. MIT Press, Cambridge, Massachusetts, pp. 165–183.

Heyes, C. and Huber, L. (eds) (2000) *The Evolution of Cognition*, MIT Press, Cambridge, Massachusetts.

Heyes, C.M. (1994) Reflections on self-recognition in primates. *Animal Behaviour* 47, 909–919.

Heyes, C.M. (1995) Self-recognition in primates: further reflections create a hall of mirrors. *Animal Behaviour* 50, 1533–1542.

Hiebert, T. (1996) *The Yahwist's Landscape: Nature and Religion in Early Israel*. Oxford University Press, Oxford, UK.

Hill, S.P. and Broom, D.M. (2009) Measuring zoo animal welfare: theory and practice. *Zoo Biology* 28, 531–544.

Hinde, R.A. (1970) *Animal Behaviour: A Synthesis of Ethology and Comparative Psychology*, 2nd edn. McGraw Hill, New York.

Holst, D. von (1986) Vegetative and somatic components of tree shrews' behaviour. *Journal of the Autonomic Nervous System Supplement* 1986, 657–670.

Houdebine, L.M. (2005) Use of transgenic animals to improve human health and animal production. *Reproduction in Domestic Animals* 40, 269–281.

Huber, R.C., Remuge, L., Carlisle, A., Lillico, S., Sandøe, P., Sørensen, D.B., Whitelaw, C.B.A. and Olsson, I.A.S. (2012) Welfare assessment in transgenic pigs expressing green fluorescent protein (GFP). *Transgenic Research* 21, 773–784.

Hughes, B.O. (1982) The historical and ethical background of animal welfare. In: Uglow, J. (ed.) *How Well do Our Animals Fare?* Proceedings of the 15th Annual Conference of the Reading University Agricultural Club 1981, pp. 1–9.

Hughes, B.O. and Black, A.J. (1973) The preference of domestic hens for different types of battery cage floor. *British Poultry Science* 14, 615–619.

Hughes, B.O. and Duncan, I.J.H. (1988) Behavioural needs: can they be explained in terms of motivational models? *Applied Animal Behaviour Science* 20, 352–355.

Hughes, B.O., Hughes, G.S., Waddington, D. and Appleby, M.C. (1996) Behavioural comparison of transgenic and control sheep: movement order, behaviour on pasture and in covered pens. *Animal Science* 63, 91–101.

Humphrey, N.K. (1986) *The Inner Eye*. Faber and Faber, London.

Humphrey, N.K. (1992) *A History of Mind*. Chatto and Windus, London.

Huntingford, F.A., Adams, C., Braithwaite, V.A., Kadri, S., Pottinger, T.G., Dandoe, P. and Turnbull, J.F. (2006) Current issues in fish welfare. *Journal of Fish Biology* 68, 332–372.

Hutson, G.D. (1989) Operant tests of access to earth as a reinforcement for weaner piglets. *Animal Production* 48, 561–569.

Huttenlocher, P.R. (1993) Morphometric study of human cerebral cortex development. In: Johnson, M.H. (ed.) *Brain Development and Cognition*. Blackwell, Oxford, UK, pp. 112–124.

Iggo, A. (1984) *Pain in Animals*. Universities Federation for Animal Welfare, Potters Bar, UK.

Iriki, A., Tanaka, M., Obayashi, S. and Iwamura, Y. (2001) Self-images in the video monitor coded by monkey intraparietal neurons. *Neuroscience Research* 40, 163–173.

Itakura, S. and Imamizu, H. (1994) An explanatory study of mirror-image shape-discrimination in young children – vision and touch. *Perceptual and Motor Skills* 78, 83–88.

Jackson, C. (2003) Laboratory fish: impacts of pain and stress on well-being. *Contemporary Topics* 42, 62–73.

Jackson, N.W. and Elwood, R.W. (1989) Memory of shells in the hermit crab, *Pagurus bernhardus*. *Animal Behaviour* 37, 529–534.

Jackson, R.R. and Cross, F.R. (2011) Spider cognition. *Advances in Insect Physiology* 41, 115–174.

Jackson, R.R. and Wilcox, R.S. (1994) Spider flexibly chooses aggressive mimicry signals for different prey by trial and error. *Behaviour* 127, 21–36.

Jensen, P. (1986) Observations on the maternal behaviour of free ranging domestic pigs. *Applied Animal Behaviour Science* 16, 131–142.

Jerison, H.J. (1973) *Evolution of Brain and Intelligence*. Academic Press, New York.

Johnson, M.H. (1993) Cerebral maturation and the development of visual attention in early infancy. In: Johnson, M.H. (ed.) *Brain Development and Cognition*. Blackwell, Oxford, UK, pp. 167–194.

Jolly, A. (1966) Lemur social behaviour and primate intelligence. *Science, New York* 153, 501–506.

Kaminski, J., Tempelmann, S., Call, J. and Tomasello, M. (2009) Domestic dogs comprehend human communication with iconic signs. *Developmental Science* 12, 831–837.

Kavaliers, M. (1989) Evolutionary aspects of the neuromodulation of nociceptive behaviors. *American Zoologist* 29, 1345–1353.

Kavaliers, M. and Hirst, M. (1983) Tolerance to morphine-induced thermal response in the terrestrial snail, *Cepaea nemoralis*. *Neuropharmacology* 22, 1321–1326.

Kawai, N., Kono, R. and Sugimoto, S. (2004) Avoidance learning in the crayfish (*Procambarus clarkii*) depends on the predatory imminence of the unconditioned stimulus: a behavior systems approach to learning in invertebrates. *Behavioural Brain Research* 150, 229–237.

Keeling, L. and Jensen, P. (2002) Behavioural disturbances, stress and welfare. In: Jensen, P. (ed.) *The Ethology of Domestic Animals*. CAB International, Wallingford, UK, pp. 79–98.

Keeling, L.J. (2005) Healthy and happy: animal welfare as an integral part of sustainable agriculture. *AMBIO* 34, 316–319.

Keenan, J.P., Gallup, G.G. and Falk, D. (2003) *The Face in the Mirror: The Search for the Origins of Consciousness*. Harper Collins, New York.

Kendrick, K.M. and Baldwin, B.A. (1987) Cells in the temporal cortex of sheep can respond preferentially to the sight of faces. *Science, NewYork* 236, 448–450.

Kendrick, K.M., Atkins, K., Hinton, M.R., Borad, K.D., Fabre-Nys, C. and Keverne, B. (1995) Facial and vocal discrimination in sheep. *Animal Behaviour* 49, 1665–1676.

Kendrick, K.M., da Costa, A.P., Leigh, A.E., Hinton, M.R. and Peirce, J.W. (2001) Sheep don't forget a face. *Nature* 414, 165–166.

Kilgour, R. (1987) Learning and the training of farm animals. In: Price, E.O. (ed.) *The Veterinary Clinics of North America, Vol. 3, No. 2, Farm Animal Behavior.* Veterinary Clinics of North America, Philadelphia, Pennsylvania.

Kirkden, R.D., Edwards, J.S.S. and Broom, D.M. (2003) A theoretical comparison of the consumer surplus and the elasticities of demand as measures of motivational strength. *Animal Behaviour* 65, 157–178.

Kirkwood, J.K. (2006) The distribution of the capacity for sentience in the animal kingdom. In: Turner, J. and D'Silva, J. (eds) *Animals, Ethics and Trade: The Challenge of Animal Sentience.* Compassion in World Farming Trust, Petersfield, UK, pp. 12–26.

Knierim, U., Carter, C.S., Fraser, D., Gärtner, K., Lutgendorf, S.K., Mineka, S., Panksepp, J. and Sachser, N. (2001) Group report: good welfare: improving quality of life. In: Broom, D.M. (ed.) *Coping with Challenge: Welfare in Animals Including Humans.* Dahlem University Press, Berlin, pp. 79–100.

Knowles, T.G. and Broom, D.M. (1990) Limb-bone strength and movement in laying hens from different housing systems. *Veterinary Record* 14, 354–356.

Koolhaas, J.M., Korte, S.M., de Boer, S.F., van de Vegt, B.A., van Reenen, C.G. and Hopster, H. (1999) Coping styles in animals: current status in behavior and stress physiology. *Neuroscience Biobehavioral Review* 23, 925–935.

Kropotkin, R. (1902) *Mutual Aid: A Factor in Evolution.* Allen Lane, London.

Kummer, H. (1978) Analogs of morality among non-human primates. In: Stent, G.S. (ed.) *Morality as a Biological Phenomenon.* University of California Press, Berkeley and Los Angeles, California, pp. 31–47.

Laming, P.R. (ed.) (1981) *Brain Mechanisms of Behaviour in Lower Vertebrates.* Cambridge University Press, Cambridge, UK.

Langbein, J., Nürnberg, G. and Manteuffel, G. (2004) Visual discrimination learning in dwarf goats and associated changes in heart rate and heart rate variability. *Physiology and Behavior* 82, 601–609.

Leach, M.C., Klaus, K., Miller, A.L., di Perrotolo, M.S., Sotocinal, S.G. and Flecknell, P.A. (2012) The assessment of post-vasectomy pain in mice using behaviour and the mouse grimace scale. *PLoS ONE* 7, e35656.

Leavens, D.A. (2007) Animal cognition: multimodal tactics of orang-utan communication. *Current Biology* 17, R762–R764.

Le Doux, J.E. (1995) Emotion: clues from the brain. *Annual Review of Psychology* 46, 209–235.

Lee, B.H. (2002) Managing pain in human neonates – applications for animals. *Journal of the American Veterinary Medical Association* 221, 233–237.

Lee, P.C. (1999) *Comparative Primate Socioecology.* Cambridge University Press, Cambridge, UK.

Lee, S.J., Ralston, H.J.P., Partridge, J.C. and Rosen, M.A. (2005) Fetal pain: a systematic multidisciplinary review of the evidence. *Journal of the American Medical Association* 294, 947–954.

Lefebre, L., Whittle, P., Lascaris, E. and Finkelstein, A. (1997) Feeding innovations and forebrain size in birds. *Animal Behaviour* 53, 549–560.

Lewis, M. and Brooks-Guy, J. (1979) *Social Cognition and the Acquisition of Self.* Plenum, New York.

Lloyd, J.E. (1986) Firefly communication and deception, oh what a tangled web! In: Mitchell, R.W. and Thompson, N.S. (eds) *Deception.* SUNY Press, Albany, New York, pp. 113–128.

Lloyd Morgan, C. (1896) *Habit and Instinct.* Edward Arnold, London.

Lohmann, K.J., Pentcheff, N.D., Nevitt, G.A., Stetten, G.D., Zimmerfaust, R.K., Jarrard, H.E. and Boles, L.C. (1995) Magnetic orientation of spiny lobsters in the ocean: experiments with undersea coil systems. *Journal of Experimental Biology* 198, 2041–2048.

Lorenzetti, F.D., Mozzachiodi, R., Baxter, D.Q. and Byrne, J.H. (2006) Classical and operant conditioning differentially modify the intrinsic properties of an identified neuron. *Nature Neuroscience* 9, 17–19.

Love, J., Gribbin, C., Mather, C. and Sang, H. (1994) Transgenic birds by DNA micro-injection. *Biotechnology* 12, 60–63.

Lozda, M., Romanao, A. and Maldonado, H. (1988) Effect of morphine and naloxone on a defensive response of the crab, *Chasmagnathus granulatus. Pharmacology Biochemistry and Behavior* 30, 635–640.

Lunzer, E.A. (1979) The development of consciousness. In: Underwood, G. and Stevens, R. (eds) *Aspects of Consciousness: Vol. 1 Psychological Issues.* Academic Press, London, pp. 1–19.

Lyall, J., Irvine, R.M., Sherman, A., Mckinley, T.I., Núñez, A., Purdie, A., Outtrim, L. *et al.* (2011) Suppression of avian influenza transmission in genetically modified chickens. *Science* 331, 223–226.

Lyche, J.L., Janczak, M., Eriksen, M.S. and Braastad, B.O. (2005) Fosterets evne til å oppleve ubehag, smerte og stress. Rapport Institutt for Produksjonsdyrmedisin, Norges Veterinærhøgskole, Oslo.

Maldonado, H. and Miralto, A. (1982) Effect of morphine and naloxone on a defensive response of the mantis shrimp (*Squilla mantis*). *Journal of Comparative Physiology A* 147, 455–459.

Manser, C.E., Elliott, H., Morris, T.H. and Broom, D.M. (1996) The use of a novel operant test to determine the strength of preference for flooring in laboratory rats. *Laboratory Animals* 30, 1–6.

Manser, C.E., Broom, D.M., Overend, R. and Morris, T.H. (1998a) Investigation into the preference of laboratory rats for nest-boxes and nesting materials. *Laboratory Animals* 32, 23–35.

Manser, C.E., Broom, D.M., Overend, R. and Morris, T.H. (1998b) Operant studies to determine the strength of preference in laboratory rats for nest-boxes and nesting material. *Laboratory Animals* 32, 36–41.

Manteuffel, G., Langbein, J. and Puppe, B. (2009) From operant learning to cognitive enrich-ment in farm animal housing: bases and applicability. *Animal Welfare* 18, 87–95.

Marchant, J.N. and Broom, D.M. (1996) Effects of dry sow housing conditions on muscle weight and bone strength. *Animal Science* 62, 105–113.

Marsh, D.F., Hatch, D.J. and Fitzgerald, M. (1997) Opioid systems and the newborn. *British Journal of Anaesthesia* 79, 787–795.

Marten, K. and Psakoros, S. (1995) Using self-view television to distinguish between self-examination and social behavior in the bottlenose dolphin (*Tursiops truncatus*). *Consciousness and Cognition* 4, 205–224.

Martin, L.N. and Delgado, M.R. (2013) The neural basis of positive and negative emo-tion regulation: implications for decision making. In: Delgado, M.R., Phelps, E.A. and Robbins, T.W. (eds) *Decision Making, Affect and Learning.* Oxford University Press, Oxford, UK, pp. 311–327.

Mason, G.J., Cooper, J.J. and Clarebrough, C. (2001) Frustrations of fur-farmed mink. *Nature* 410, 35–36.

Mason, G.J., Clubb, R., Latham, N. and Vickery, S. (2007) Why and how should we use environmental enrichment to tackle stereotypic behaviour? *Applied Animal Behaviour Science* 102, 163–188.

Mason, J.W. (1968) A review of psychoendocrine research on the pituitary adrenal cortical system. *Psychosomatic Medicine* 30, 576–607.

Mason, J.W. (1971) A re-evaluation of the concept of 'non-specificity' in stress theory. *Journal of Psychiatric Research* 8, 323–333.

Mather, J.A. (1995) Cognition in cephalopods. *Advances in the Study of Behavior* 24, 316–353.

Mather, J.A. (2004) Cephalopod skin displays: from concealment to communication. In: Oller, K. and Greibel, U. (eds) *Evolution of Communication Systems.* MIT Press, Cambridge, Massachusetts, pp. 193–213.

Mather, J.A. (2013) Do cephalopods have pain and suffering. In: Kemp, T.A. van der and Lachance, M. (eds) *Animal Suffering: From Science to Law.* International Symposium. Éditions Yvon Blais, Paris.

Mather, J.A. and Anderson, R.C. (2007) Ethics and invertebrates: a cephalopod perspective. *Diseases in Aquatic Organisms* 25, 119–129.

Matthews, L.R. and Ladewig, J. (1994) Environmental requirements of pigs measured by behavioural demand functions. *Animal Behaviour* 47, 713–719.

McBride, G., Parer, I.P. and Foenander, F. (1969) The social organisation of the feral domestic fowl. *Animal Behaviour Monographs* 2, 125–181.

McFarland, D.J. and Sibly, R.M. (1975) The behavioural final common path. *Philosophical Transactions of the Royal Society B* 27, 265–293.

McGrew, W.C. and Tutin, C.E.G. (1978) Evidence for a social custom in wild chimpanzees? *Man* 13, 234–251.

McLeman, M.A., Mendl, M., Jones, R.B., White, R. and Wathes, C.M. (2005) Discrimination of conspecifics by juvenile domestic pigs, *Sus scrofa. Animal Behaviour* 70, 451–461.

Mellor, D.J. (2011) Animal emotions, behaviour and the production of positive welfare states. *New Zealand Veterinary Journal* 60, 1–8.

Mellor, D.J. and Diesch, T.J. (2006) Onset of sentience: the potential for suffering in fetal and newborn farm animals. *Applied Animal Behaviour Science* 100, 48–57.

Mellor, D.J. and Gregory, N.G. (2003) Responsiveness, behavioural arousal and awareness in fetal and newborn lambs: experimental, practical and therapeutic implications. *New Zealand Veterinary Journal* 51, 2–13.

Mellor, D.J., Diesch, T.J., Gunn, A.J. and Bennet, L. (2005) The importance of 'awareness' for understanding fetal pain. *Brain Research Reviews* 49, 455–471.

Mendl, M. and Paul, E.S. (2004) Consciousness, emotion and animal welfare: insights from cognitive science. *Animal Welfare* 13, 17–25.

Mendl, M. and Paul, E.S. (2008) Do animals live in the present? Current evidence and implications for welfare. *Applied Animal Behaviour Science* 113, 357–382.

Mendl, M., Zanella, A.J. and Broom, D.M. (1992) Physiological and reproductive correlates of behavioural strategies in female domestic pigs. *Animal Behaviour* 44, 1107–1121.

Mendl, M., Randle, K. and Pope, S. (2002) Young female pigs can discriminate individual differences in odours from conspecific urine. *Animal Behaviour* 64, 97–101.

Mendl, M., Burman, H.P., Parker, R.M.A. and Paul, E.S. (2009) Cognitive bias as an indicator of animal emotion and welfare: emerging evidence and underlying mechanisms. *Applied Animal Behaviour Science* 118, 161–181.

Mendl, M., Burman, O.H. and Paul, E.S. (2010a) An integrative and functional framework for the study of animal emotion and mood. *Proceedings of the Royal Society B: Biological Sciences* 277(1696), 2895–2904.

Mendl, M., Brooks, J., Basse, C., Burman, O., Paul, E., Blackwell, E. and Casey, R. (2010b) Dogs showing separation-related behaviour exhibit a 'pessimistic' cognitive bias. *Current Biology* 20, R839–R840.

Menzel, E.W., Savage-Rumbaugh, E.S. and Lawson, J. (1985) Chimpanzee (*Pan troglodytes*) spatial problem solving with the use of mirrors and televised equivalents of mirrors. *Journal of Comparative Psychology* 99, 211–217.

Menzel, R., Greggers, U., Smith, A., Berger, S. and Brandt, R. (2005) Honeybees navigate according to a map-like spatial memory. *Proceedings of the National Academy of Sciences* 102, 3040–3045.

Merker, B. (2007) Consciousness without a cerebral cortex: a challenge for neuroscience and medicine. *Behaviour and Brain Sciences* 30, 63–81.

Merriam Webster (2005) *The Merriam Webster English Dictionary*. Merriam Webster, Springfield, Massachusetts.

Messenger, J.B. (2001) Cephalopod chromatophores: neurobiology and natural history. *Biological Reviews* 76, 473–528.

Midgley, M. (1994) *The Ethical Primate*. Routledge, London.

Miklósi, Á., Polgárdi, R., Topál, J. and Csányi, V. (2000) Intentional behaviour in dog–human communication: experimental analysis of 'showing' behaviour in the dog. *Animal Cognition* 3, 159–166.

Miller, N.E. (1959) Liberalization of basic S-R concepts: extensions to conflict behaviour, motivation and social learning. In: Koch, S. (ed.) *Psychology: A Study of a Science, Vol. II*. McGraw Hill, New York.

Mineka, S., Watson, D. and Clark, L.A. (1998) Comorbidity of anxiety and unipolar mood disorders. *Annual Review of Psychology* 49, 377–412.

Mizunami, M., Okada, R., Li, Y. and Strausfeld, N.J. (1998) Mushroom bodies of the cockroach: activity and identitities of neurons. *Journal of Comparative Neurology* 519, 501–519.

Moberg, G.P. (1985) Biological response to stress, key to assessment of animal well-being? In: Moberg, G.P. (ed.) *Animal Stress*. American Physiological Society, Bethesda, Maryland, pp. 27–49.

Moe, R.O., Stubsjøen, S.M., Bohlin, J., Flø, A. and Bakken, M. (2012) Peripheral temperature drop in response to anticipation and consumption of a signaled palatable reward in laying hens *Gallus domesticus*. *Physiology and Behavior* 106, 527–533.

Moore, G.E. (1903) *Principia Ethica*. Cambridge University Press, Cambridge, UK.

Morton, D.B. and Griffiths, P.H.M. (1985) Guidelines on the recognition of pain, distress and discomfort in experimental animals and an hypothesis for assessment. *Veterinary Record* 116, 431–436.

Mount, L.E. (1979) *Adaptation to Thermal Environment*. Edward Arnold, London.

Moynihan, M. (1985) *Communication and Non-communication by Cephalopods*. Indiana Press, Bloomington, Indiana.

Murray, E.A. (2007) The amygdala, reward and emotion. *Trends in Cognitive Science* 11, 489–497.

Napolitano, F., De Rosa, G. and Sevi, A. (2008) Welfare implications of artificial rearing and early weaning in sheep. *Applied Animal Behaviour Science* 110, 58–72.

Neely, G.G., Keene, A.C., Duchek, P., Chang, E.C., Wang, O.-P., Aksoy, Y.A., Rosenzweig, M. *et al.* (2011) TrpA1 regulates thermal nociception in *Drosophila*. *PLoS ONE* 6, 1–9.

Nelson, E. and Panksepp, J. (1998) Brain substrates of infant–mother attachment: contributions of opioids, oxytocin and nor-epinephrine. *Neuroscience and Bio-behavioral Reviews* 22, 437–452.

Nettle, D. and Bateson, M. (2012) The evolutionary origins of mood and its disorders. *Current Biology* 22, R712–R721.

Niemann, H. and Kues, W.A. (2003) Application of transgenesis in livestock for agriculture and biomedicine. *Animal Reproduction Science* 79, 291–317.

Nixon, M. and Young, J.Z. (2003) *The Brains and Lives of Cephalopods.* Oxford University Press, Oxford, UK.

Nørgaard-Nielsen, G.J. (1990) Bone strength of laying hens kept in an alternative system compared with hens in cages and or on deep-litter. *British Poultry Science* 31, 81–89.

Odling-Smee, L. and Braithwaite, V.A. (2003) The role of learning in fish orientation. *Fish and Fisheries* 4, 235–246.

O'Flanagan, J. (1992) *Consciousness Reconsidered.* MIT Press, Cambridge, Massachusetts.

OIE (World Organisation for Animal Health) (2011) *Terrestrial Animal Health Code.* OIE, Paris.

Oltenacu, P.A. and Broom, D.M. (2010) The impact of genetic selection for increased milk yield on the welfare of dairy cows. *Animal Welfare* 19 (S), 39–49.

Ouedraogo, A. and Le Neindre, P. (1999) *L'Homme et l'Animal: Un Debat de Société.* INRA Editions, Paris.

Oxford English Dictionary (2011) *Concise Oxford English Dictionary.* Oxford University Press, Oxford, UK.

Palmiter, R.D. (1986) Germline transformation of mice. *Annual Review of Genetics* 20, 465–499.

Panksepp, J. (1998) *Affective Neuroscience. The Foundation of Human and Animal Emotion.* Oxford University Press, New York.

Panksepp, J. (2003) At the interface of the affective, behavioural and cognitive neurosciences: decoding the emotional feelings of the brain. *Brain and Cognition* 52, 4–14.

Panksepp, J. (2005) Affective consciousness: core emotional feelings in animals and humans. *Consciousness and Cognition* 14, 30–80.

Parrott, R.F., Hall, S.J.G., Lloyd, D.M., Goode, J.A. and Broom, D.M. (1998) Effects of a maximum permissible journey time (31h) on physiological responses of fleeced and shorn sheep to transport, with observations on behaviour during a short (1h) rest-stop. *Animal Science* 66, 197–207.

Paton, M.W. and Martin, P.A.J. (2006) Can composite indices and risk assessment be used to evaluate animal welfare. *Proceedings of the 11th International Symposium on Veterinary and Economics.* Sci-quest, New Zealand, p. 375.

Paul, E.S., Harding, E.J. and Mendl, M. (2005) Measuring emotional processes in animals: the utility of a cognitive approach. *Neuroscience and Biobehavioral Reviews* 29, 469–491.

Pepperberg, I.M. (2000) *The Alex Studies: Cognitive and Communicative Abilities of Grey Parrots.* Harvard University Press, Cambridge, Massachusetts.

Perry, S. and Bernier, N.J. (1999) The acute hormonal adrenergic stress response in fish: facts and fiction. *Aquaculture* 177, 285–295.

Phillips, C.J.C. and Santurtun, E. (2013) The welfare of livestock transported by ship. *The Veterinary Journal* 196, 309–314.

Phillips, M.L., Bullmore, E.T., Howard, R., Woodruff, P.W., Wright, I.C., Williams, S.C.R., Simmons, A. *et al.* (1998) Investigation of facial recognition memory and happy and sad facial expression perception: an fMRI study. *Psychiatry Research: Neuroimaging* 83, 127–138.

Planalp, S. (1999) *Communicating Emotion: Social, Moral and Cultural Processes.* Cambridge University Press, Cambridge, UK and Maisons des Sciences de l'Homme, Paris.

Plotnik, J.M., Waal, F.B.M. de and Reiss, D. (2006) Self-recognition in an Asian elephant. *Proceedings of the National Academy of Sciences* 103, 17053–17057.

Pollan, M. (2006) *The Omnivore's Dilemma: A Natural History of Four Meals.* Penguin Books, London.

Pongrácz, P., Miklósi, A., Vida, V. and Csányi, V. (2005) The pet dog's ability for learning from a human demonstrator in a detour task is independent of breed and age. *Applied Animal Behaviour Science* 90, 309–323.

Portavella, M., Torres, B. and Salas, C. (2004) Avoidance response in goldfish: emotional and temporal involvement of medial and lateral telencephatic pallium. *Journal of Neuroscience* 24, 2335–2342.

Povinelli, D.J., Landau, K.R. and Perilloux, H.K. (1996) Self-recognition in young children using delayed versus live feedback: evidence of a developmental asynchrony. *Child Development* 67, 1540–1554.

Price, E.O. (2002) *Animal Domestication and Behaviour.* CAB International, Wallingford, UK.

Prior, H., Schwarz, A. and Güntürken, O. (2008) Mirror-induced behavior in the magpie (*Pica pica*): evidence of self recognition. *PLoS Biology* 6(8), e202.doi:10.137 journal.

Pruitt, J.N., Iturralde, G., Avilés, L. and Riechert, S.L. (2011) Amazonian social spiders share similar within-colony behavioral variation and behavioral syndromes. *Animal Behaviour* 82, 1449–1455.

Raby, C.R. and Clayton, N.S. (2009) Prospective cognition in animals. *Behavioural Processes* 80, 314–324.

Raby, C.R., Alexis, D.M., Dickinson, A. and Clayton, N.S. (2007) Planning for the future by western scrub jays. *Nature* 445, 919–921.

Radford, M. (2001) *Animal Welfare Law in Britain: Regulation and Responsibility.* Oxford University Press, Oxford, UK.

Reader, S.M. and Laland, K.N. (2002) Social intelligence, innovation, and enhanced brain size in primates. *Proceedings of the National Academy of Sciences* 99, 4436–4441.

Reader, S.M. and Laland, K.N. (2003) *Animal Innovation.* Oxford University Press, Oxford, UK.

Redwine, I.S., Altemus, M., Leong, Y.-M. and Cater, C.S. (2001) Lymphocyte responses to stress in post partum women: relationship to vagal tone. *Psychoneuroendocrinology* 26, 241–251.

Reese, E.S. (1989) Orientation behaviour of butterfly fishes (family Chaetodontidae) on coral reefs – spatial learning of route specific landmarks and cognitive maps. *Environmental Biology of Fishes* 25, 79–86.

Regan, T. (1990) Animal rights. In: Clarke, S.R.L. and Linzey, A. (eds) *Political Theory and Animal Rights.* Pluto Press, London, pp. 176–186.

Regolin, L., Vallortigara, G. and Zanforlin, M. (1995) Object and spatial representations in detour problems by chicks. *Animal Behaviour* 49, 195–199.

Reid, P.J. (2009) Adapting to the human world: dogs' responsiveness to our social cues. *Behavioural Processes* 80, 325–333.

Reiss, D. and Marino, L. (2001) Mirror self-recognition in the bottle nose dolphin: a cased cognitive consequence. *Proceedings of the National Academy of Sciences* 98, 5937–5942.

Reznikova, Z.A. (2003) Government and nepotism in social insects: new dimension provided by an experimental approach. *Eurasian Entomology Journal* 2, 1–12.

Reznikova, Z.A. (2007) *Animal Intelligence: From Individual to Social Cognition*. Cambridge University Press, Cambridge, UK.

Ridley, M. (1996) *The Origins of Virtue*. Viking, London.

Robertson, J.D., Bonaventura, J. and Kohm, A. (1995) Nitric-oxide synthetase inhibition blocks octopus touch learning without producing sensor or motor dysfunction. *Proceedings of the Royal Society of London Series B – Biological Sciences* 261, 167–172.

Robertson, S.S. (1987) Human cyclic motility: fetal-newborn continuities and newborn state difference. *Developmental Psychobiology* 20, 425–442.

Robinson, S.R. and Smotherman, W.P. (1992) The amniotic sac as scaffolding: prenatal ontogeny of an action plan. *Developmental Psychobiology* 24, 463–485.

Rochat, P. (2002) Origins of self concept. In: Bremner, J.G. and Fogel, A. (eds) *Blackwell Handbook of Infant Development*. Blackwell, Oxford, UK.

Rochat, P. and Striano, T. (2002) Who's in the mirror? Self-other discrimination in specular images by four- and nine-month-old infants. *Child Development* 73, 35–46.

Rodriguez, F., Duran, E., Vargas, J.P., Torres, B. and Salas, C. (1994) Performance of goldfish trained in allocentric and egocentric maze procedures suggests the presence of a cognitive mapping system in fishes. *Animal Learning and Behaviour* 22, 409–420.

Rodriguez-Moldes, I., Manso, M.J., Becerra, M., Molist, P. and Anadon, R. (1993) Distribution of substance P-like immunoreactivity in the brain of the elasmobranch *Scyliorhinus canicula*. *Journal of Comparative Neurology* 333, 228–244.

Rollin, B.E. (1989) *The Unheeded Cry: Animal Consciousness, Animal Pain and Science*. Oxford University Press, Oxford, UK.

Rollin, B.E. (1995) *Farm Animal Welfare: Social, Bioethical and Research Issues*. Iowa State University Press, Ames, Iowa.

Rolls, E.T. (1999) *The Brain and Emotion*. Oxford University Press, Oxford, UK.

Rolls, E.T. (2005) *Emotion Explained*. Oxford University Press, Oxford, UK.

Rooijakkers, E.F., Kaminski, J. and Call, J. (2009) Comparing dogs and great apes in their ability to visually track object transpositions. *Animal Cognition* 12, 789–796.

Rooijen, J. van (1980) Wahlversuche, eine ethologische Methode zum Sammeln von Messwerten, un Haltungseinflusse zu erfassen und zu beurteilen. *Aktuelle Arbeiten zur artgemässen Tierhaltung, K.T.B.L.-Schrift* 264, 165–185.

Rosati, A., Stevens, J., Hare, B. and Hauser, M. (2007) The evolutionary origins of human patience: temporal preferences in chimpanzees, bonobos and human adults. *Current Biology* 17, 1663–1668.

Rose, J.D. (2002) The neurobehavioral nature of fishes and the question of awareness and pain. *Reviews in Fisheries Science* 10, 1–38.

Ross, L.G. and Ross, B. (2009) *Anaesthetic and Sedative Techniques for Aquatic Animals*, 3rd edn. Blackwell, Oxford, UK.

Rossi, A.P. and Ades, C. (2008) A dog at the keyboard: using arbitrary signs to communicate requests. *Animal Cognition* 11, 329–338.

Rousing, T. and Wemelsfelder, F. (2006) Qualitative assessment of social behaviour of dairy cows housed in loose housing systems. *Applied Animal Behaviour Science* 101, 40–53.

Rowlands, M. (2012) *Can Animals be Moral?* Oxford University Press, New York.

Rowlands, M. (2013) *Running with the Pack*. Granta Books, London.

Rugani, R., Fontanari, L., Simoni, E., Regolin, L. and Vallortigara, G. (2009) Arithmetic in newborn chicks. *Proceedings of the Royal Society B*, 276, 2451–2460.

Rumbaugh, D.M., Beran, M.J. and Hillix, W.A. (2000) Cause-effect reasoning in humans and animals. In: Heyes, C. and Huber, L. (eds) *The Evolution of Cognition*. MIT Press, Cambridge, Massachusetts, pp. 221–238.

Rushen, J. (1986) Aversion of sheep for handling treatments: paired-choice experiments. *Applied Animal Behaviour Science* 16, 363–370.

Russell, W.M.S. and Burch, R.L. (1959) *The Principles of Humane Animal Experimentation Technique*. Methuen, London.

Ryan, Y.M. (1997) Meat avoidance and body weight concerns : nutritional implications for teenage girls. *Proeedings of the Nutrition Society* 56, 519–524.

Sandeman, D., Sandeman, R., Derby, C. and Schmidt, M. (1992) Morphology of the brain of crayfish, crabs, and spiny lobsters: a common nomenclature for homologous structures. *Biological Bulletin* 183, 304–326.

Sander, D. (2013) Models of emotion: the affective neuroscience approach. In: Armony, J. and Vuilleumier, P. (eds) *The Cambridge Handbook of Affective Neuroscience*. Cambridge University Press, Cambridge, UK, pp. 5–53.

Sapontzis, S.F. (1987) *Morals, Reason and Animals*. Temple University Press, Philadelphia, Pennsylvania.

Schaik, C.P. van, Damerius, L. and Isler, K. (2013) Wild orangutan males plan and communicate their travel direction one day in advance. *PLoS ONE* 8(9), e74896, pp. 10.

Scherer, K.R. (1999) Appraisal theories. In: Dalgleish, T. and Power, M. (eds) *Handbook of Cognition and Emotion*. Wiley, Chichester, UK, pp. 637–663.

Schjolden, J., Stoskhus, S. and Winberg, S. (2005) Does individual variation in stress responses and agonistic behavior reflect divergent stress coping strategies in juvenile rainbow trout? *Physiology Biochemistry and Zoology* 78, 715–723.

Serpell, J.A. (1986) *In the Company of Animals*. Cambridge University Press, Cambridge, UK.

Serpell, J.A. (1989) Attitudes to animals. In: Paterson, D. and Palmer, M. (eds) *The Status of Animals: Ethics Education and Welfare*. CAB International, Wallingford, UK, pp. 162–166.

Serpell, J. and Paul, E. (1994) Pets and the development of positive attitudes to animals. In: Manning, A. and Serpell, J. (eds) *Animals and Human Society*. Routledge, London, pp. 127–144.

Seth, A.K. and Baars, B.J. (2004) Neural Darwinism and consciousness. *Consciousness and Cognition* 14, 140–168.

Seth, A.K., Baars, B.J. and Edelman, D.B. (2005) Criteria for consciousness in humans and other mammals. *Consciousness and Cognition* 14, 119–139.

Sherwin, C.M. (2001) Can invertebrates suffer? Or, how robust is argument-by-analogy? *Animal Welfare* 10 (Suppl.), S103–S118.

Shettleworth, S.J. (1998) *Cognition, Evolution and Behavior*. Oxford University Press, Oxford, UK.

Shettleworth, S.J. (2009) *Cognition, Evolution and Behavior*, 2nd edn. Oxford University Press, Oxford, UK.

Shutt, D.A., Fell, L.R., Cornell, R., Bell, A.K., Wallace, C.A. and Smith, A.I. (1987) Stress-induced changes in plasma concentrations of immunoreactive β-endorphin and cortisol in response to routine surgical procedures in lambs. *Australian Journal of Biological Science* 40, 97–103.

Simons, J.P., Wilmut, I., Clark, A.J., Archibald, A.L., Bishop, J.O. and Lathe, R. (1998) Gene transfer into sheep. *Biotechnology* 6, 171–183.

Singer, P. (1994) *Ethics*. Oxford University Press, Oxford, UK.

Smith, J.D., Shields, W.E. and Washburn, D.A. (2003) The comparative psychology of uncertainty monitoring and metacognition. *Behavioral and Brain Sciences* 26, 317–339.

Smith, K.A. and Boyd, K.M. (1991) *Lives in the Balance: The Ethics of Using Animals in Biomedical Research*. Oxford University Press, Oxford, UK.

Smulders, F.J.M. and Algers, B. (eds) (2009) *Welfare of Production Animals: Assessment and Management of Risks*. Wageningen Academic Publishers, Wageningen, Netherlands.

Sneddon, L.U. (2002) Anatomical and electrophysiological analysis of the trigeminal nerve in a teleost fish, *Oncorhynchus mykiss*. *Neuroscience Letters* 319, 167–171.

Sneddon, L.U., Braithwaite, V.A. and Gentle, M.J. (2003a) Do fish have nociceptors? Evidence for the evolution of a vertebrate sensory system. *Proceedings of the Royal Society of London B* 270, 1115–1121.

Sneddon, L.U., Braithwaite, V.A. and Gentle, M.J. (2003b) Novel object test: examining nociception and fear in the rainbow trout. *Journal of Pain* 4, 431–440.

Snyder, A., Bossomaier, T. and Mitchell, D.J. (2004) Concept formation: object attributes dynamically inhibited from conscious awareness. *Journal of Integrative Neuroscience* 3, 31–46.

Sommerville, B.A. and Broom, D.M. (1998) Olfactory awareness. *Applied Animal Behaviour Science* 57, 269–286.

Sommerville, B.A., Settle, R.H., Darling, F.M.C. and Broom, D.M. (1993) The use of trained dogs to discriminate human scent. *Animal Behaviour* 46, 189–190.

Sorabji, R. (1993) *Animal Minds and Human Morals: The Origins of the Western Debate*. Cornell University Press, Ithaca, New York.

Sovrano, V.A. and Bisazza, A. (2003) Modularity as a fish (*Zenotoca eisen*) views it: conjoining and non-geometric information for special reorientations. *Journal of Experimental Psychology* 29, 199–210.

Spruijt, B.M., van den Bos, R. and Pijlman, F.T.A. (2001) A concept of welfare based on reward evaluating mechanisms in the brain: anticipatory behaviour as an indicator of the state of reward systems. *Applied Animal Behaviour Science* 75, 145–171.

Stafford, K.J., Mellor, D.J., Todd, S.E., Ward, R.N. and McMeekan, C.M. (2003) The effect of different combinations of lignocaine, ketoprophen, xylazine and tolazoline on the acute cortisol response to dehorning in calves. *New Zealand Veterinary Journal* 51, 219–226.

Stefano, G.B., Salzet, B. and Fricchione, G.L. (1998) Enkelytin and opioid peptide association in invertebrates and vertebrates: immune activation and pain. *Immunology Today* 19, 265–268.

Stefano, G.B., Cadet, P., Zhu, W., Rialas, C.M., Mantione, K., Benz, D., Fuentes, R. *et al.* (2002) The blueprint for stress can be found in invertebrates. *Neuroendocrinology Letters* 23, 85–93.

Stilwell, G., Lima, M.S. and Broom, D.M. (2008) Effects of nonsteroidal anti-inflammatory drugs on long-term pain in calves castrated by use of an external clamping technique following epidural anaesthesia. *American Journal of Veterinary Research* 69, 744–750.

Stolba, A. and Wood-Gush, D.G.M. (1989) The behaviour of pigs in a semi-natural environment. *Animal Production* 48, 419–425.

Suits, B. (1967) What is a game? *Philosophy of Science* 34, 148–156.

Suits, B. (2005) *The Grasshopper: Games, Life and Utopia*. Broadview Press, Peterborough, Ontario, Canada.

Sumpter, J.P. (1997) The endocrinology of stress. In: Iwama, G.K., Pickering, A.D., Sumpter, J.P. and Schreck, C.B. (eds) *Fish Stress and Health in Aquaculture*. Cambridge University Press, Cambridge, UK, pp. 95–118.

Swaney, W., Kendal, J., Capon, H., Brown, C. and Laland, K.N. (2001) Familiarity facilitates social learning of foraging behaviour in the guppy. *Animal Behaviour* 62, 591–598.

Tan, J. and Hare, B. (2013) Bonobos share with strangers. *PLoS ONE* 8, E51922, 1–11.

Tarsitano, M.S. and Jackson, R.R. (1994) Jumping spiders make predatory detours requiring movement away from prey. *Behaviour* 131, 65–73.

Tarsitano, M.S. and Jackson, R.R. (1997) Araneophagic jumping spiders discriminate between detour routes that do and do not lead to prey. *Animal Behaviour* 53, 257–266.

Taylor, A.H., Hunt, G.R., Holzhalder, J.C. and Gray, R.D. (2007) Spontaneous metatool use by New Caledonian crows. *Current Biology* 17, 1504–1507.

Terrace, H.S. (1984) Animal cognition. In: Roitblat, H.L., Bever, T.G. and Terrace, H.S. (eds) *Animal Cognition*. Erlbaum, Hillsdale, New Jersey, pp. 7–28.

Thorpe, W.H. (1965) The assessment of pain and distress in animals. Appendix III in *Report of the Technical Committee to Enquire into the Welfare of Animals Kept Under Intensive Husbandry Conditions*. F.W.R. Brambell (chairman). HMSO, London.

Toates, F. (2002) Physiology, motivation and the organization of behaviour. In: Jensen, P. (ed.) *The Ethology of Domestic Animals*. CAB International, Wallingford, UK, pp. 31–50.

Toates, F. and Jensen, P. (1991) Ethological and psychological models of motivation: towards a synthesis. In: Meyer, J.A. and Wilson, S. (eds) *Farm Animals to Animats*. MIT Press, Cambridge, Massachusetts, pp. 194–205.

Tomasello, M. (2000) Two hypotheses about primate cognition. In: Heyes, C. and Huber, L. (eds) *The Evolution of Cognition*. MIT Press, Cambridge, Massachusetts, pp. 165–183.

Tomsic, D., Dimant, B. and Maldonado, H. (1996) Age-related deficits of long-term memory in the crab *Chasmagnathus*. *Journal of Comparative Physiology A* 178, 139–146.

Torres-Pereira, C. and Broom, D.M. (2010) Behavioural and emotional responses in pet dogs during performance of an obedience task in the absence of the owner. *Proceedings of the 44th Congress of the International Society for Applied Ethology*. Wageningen Academic Publishers, Wageningen, Netherlands, p. 144.

Trivers, R. (1985) *Social Evolution*. Benjamin Cummings, Menlo Park, California.

Tuyttens, F.A.M., de Graaf, S., Heerkens, J.L.T., Jacobs, L., Nalon, E., Ott, S., Stadig, L., Van Laer, E. and Ampe, B. (2014) Observer bias in animal behaviour research: can we believe what we score, if we score what we believe? *Animal Behaviour* 90, 273–280.

Tye, M. (2000) *Consciousness, Colour and Environment*. MIT Press, Cambridge, Massachusetts.

Verheijen, F.J. and Buwalda, R.J.A. (1988) *Do Pain and Fear Make a Hooked Carp in Play Suffer?* CIP – Gegevens, Utrecht, Netherlands.

Vestergaard, K. (1980) The regulation of dust-bathing and other behaviour patterns in the laying hen: a Lorenzian approach. In: Moss, R. (ed.) *The Laying Hen and its Environment. Current Topics in Veterinary Medicine and Animal Science* 8. Martinus Nijhoff, The Hague, pp. 101–113.

Vince, M.A. (1973) Effects of external stimulation on the onset of lung ventilation and the time of hatching in the fowl, duck and goose. *British Poultry Science* 14, 389–401.

Waal, F. de (1989) Food sharing and reciprocal obligations among chimpanzees. *Journal of Human Evolution* 18, 433–459.

Waal, F. de (1996) *Good Natured*. Harvard University Press, Cambridge, Massachusetts.

Wall, P.D. (1992) Defining 'pain in animals'. In: Short, C.E. and van Poznak, A. (eds) *Animal Pain*. Churchill Livingstone, New York, pp. 63–79.

Walsh, P.T., Hansell, M., Borello, W.D. and Healy, S.D. (2013) Are elaborate bird nests built using simple rules? *Avian Biology Research* 6, 157–162.

Walters, E.T. and Moroz, L.L. (2009) Molluscan memory of injury: evolutionary insights into chronic pain and neurological disorders. *Brain Behavior Evolution* 74, 206–218.

Webster, J. (2010) Sentience and animal protection. In: Bekoff, M. (ed.) *Encyclopedia of Animal Rights and Animal Welfare*, 2nd edn. Greenwood Press, Santa Barbara, California, pp. 507–511.

Weiskrantz, L. (1997) *Consciousness Lost and Found: A Neuropsychological Exploration*. Oxford University Press, Oxford, UK.

Weiss, J.M. (1971) Effects of coping behaviour in different warning signal conditions on stress pathology in rats. *Journal of Comparative and Physiological Psychology* 77, 1–13.

Welfare Quality (2009a) *Welfare Quality Assessment Protocol for Cattle*. Welfare Quality Consortium, Lelystad, Netherlands.

Welfare Quality (2009b) *Welfare Quality Assessment Protocol for Pigs*. Welfare Quality Consortium, Lelystad, Netherlands.

Welfare Quality (2009c) *Welfare Quality Assessment Protocol for Poultry*. Welfare Quality Consortium, Lelystad, Netherlands.

Wemelsfelder, F., Hunter, E.A., Mendl, M.T. and Lawrence, A.B. (2000) The spontaneous qualitative assessment of behavioural expressions in pigs: first explorations of a novel methodology for integrative animal welfare measurement. *Applied Animal Behaviour Science* 67, 193–215.

Wemelsfelder, F., Nevison, I. and Lawrence, A.B. (2009) The effect of perceived environmental background on qualitative assessments of pig behaviour. *Animal Behaviour* 78, 477–484.

Wheeler, M.B. (2003) Production of transgenic livestock: promise fulfilled. *Journal of Animal Science* 81 (Suppl. 3), 32–37.

Whiten, A. and Byrne, R.W. (1988) Tactical deception in primates. *Behavioral and Brain Sciences* 11, 233–273.

Whiten, A. and Byrne, R.W. (eds) (1997) *Machiavellian Intelligence II Extensions and Evaluations*. Cambridge University Press, Cambridge, UK.

Whiten, A., Goodall, J., McGrew, W.C., Nishida, T., Reynolds, V., Sugiyama, Y., Tutin, C.E.G. *et al.* (2001) Charting cultural variation in chimpanzees. *Behaviour* 138, 1481–1516.

WHO (World Health Organization) (1948) *Preamble to the Constitution of the World Health Organization*. Official Records of the World Health Organization 2. WHO, Geneva, Switzerland, p. 100.

Widowski, T.M. and Duncan, I.J.H. (2000) Working for a dustbath: are hens increasing pleasure rather than reducing suffering? *Applied Animal Behaviour Science* 68, 39–53.

Wilcox, R.S. and Jackson, R.R. (1998) Cognitive abilities of araneophagic jumping spiders. In: Pepperberg, I., Balda, R. and Kamil, A. (eds) *Animal Cognition in Nature*. Academic Press, San Diego, California, pp. 411–433.

Wilkinson, A., Kuenstner, K. and Huber, L. (2010) Social learning in a non-social reptile (*Geochelone carbonaria*). *Biology Letters* 6, 614–616.

Williams, G.C. (1988) Reply to comments on 'Huxley's evolution and ethics in socio-biological perspective'. *Zygon* 23, 437–438.

Wilson, E.O. (1975) *Sociobiology*. Belknap Press, Cambridge, Massachusetts.

Wood-Gush, D.G.M., Duncan, I.J.H. and Savory, C.J. (1978) Observations on the social behaviour of domestic fowl in the wild. *Biology of Behaviour* 3, 193–205.

Woolf, C.J. and Walters, E.T. (1991) Common patterns of plasticity leading to noci-ceptive sensitization in mammals and *Aplysia*. *Trend in Neuroscience* 14, 74–78.

World Trade Organization (2013) Dispute DS400 European Communities – Measures Prohibiting the Importation and Marketing of Seal Products. www.wto.org/english/tratop_e/dispu_e/cases_e/ds400_e.htm (accessed 24 March 2014).

Würbel, H. (2009) Ethology applied to animal ethics. *Applied Animal Behaviour Science* 118, 118–127.

Young, J.Z. (1991) Computation in the learning-system of cephalopods. *Biological Bulletin* 180, 200–208.

Yue, S., Moccia, R.D. and Duncan, I.J.H. (2004) Investigating fear in domestic rainbow trout, *Oncorhynchus mykiss*, using an avoidance learning task. *Applied Animal Behaviour Science* 87, 343–354.

Zaccone, G., Fasula, S. and Ainis, L. (1994) Distribution patterns of the paraneuronal endocrine cells in the skin, gills and the airways of fishes determined by immuno-histochemical and histological methods. *Histochemistry Journal* 26, 609–629.

Zimmerman, P.H., Lundberg, A., Keeling, L.J. and Koene, P. (2003) The effect of an audi-ence on the gakel call and other frustration behaviours in the laying hen (*Gallus gallus domesticus*). *Animal Welfare* 12, 315–326.

Author Index

Subject Index

aberrant behaviour Glossary, 91
abnormal behaviour Glossary, 91,
    95–97, 102–103, 113
abstract thought 42, 51, 82
adaptation Glossary, 31, 32–33, 85
adrenal 25, 32, 60–61, 79, 91–92,
    97, 140
    indicators 60, 79, 91–92
adrenaline 61
adrenocorticotrophic hormone
    (ACTH) 61, 103
aesthetics and animal treatment 14, 19,
    117, 129
affect Glossary, 52–53, 57–59, 63, 72
affection 12, 57, 69, 128
aggression Glossary, 10, 17, 96
allogrooming Glossary, 10
altricial 109–110
altruism 8–11
American Veterinary Medical
    Association 30, 34, 57, 130
amygdala 41, 60–63, 68–69, 103
anaesthesia 67, 75, 115, 121
analgesia 67, 99, 115, 121
anger 57–58, 68 –69
animal, biological meaning ix, 5
animal husbandry 28, 119, 121, 140
Animal Machines 24, 137
animal production 6, 18, 20, 24, 26, 31,
    56, 125–128, 131, 132, 135,
    136–139
animal protection 4, 15, 21, 24, 29, 36,
    64, 109, 116–117, 119 –120,
    122–123, 138–140

animal rights 14–17, 24, 120
animal training 20, 41, 79
animal welfare 4, 9, 14–15, 22–36,
    90–107, 126–155
    journals 20, 26
    teaching 19–20, 30, 140
Animal Welfare Science Hub 140
ant 46, 49, 119
anti-predator behaviour 11, 35, 39, 47,
    50, 65, 67, 73, 74, 78, 98–100, 102
anxiety 3, 15, 52, 63, 65, 68
Aplysia 40, 49, 66–67, 72, 129
arousal 68, 111
ascites 131
attitudes to animals 18–21
aversion 64, 93
aversive Glossary, 5, 40, 62
avoidance 15, 35, 47, 49, 55–56,
    64–67, 74, 77, 99
awareness Glossary, 2, 3, 5, 6, 19, 29,
    39, 40, 42, 44, 46, 47, 51,
    55, 59–60, 72–83, 109–113,
    118–119
    degree of 5, 55, 64, 120, 122
    evolution of 49, 83
    of others 19, 51, 77–78, 82–83
    of self 19, 46, 55, 78, 80–81

baboon 50
barren environment 27
battery cage 96, 139
beak-trimming 121
bee 122, 129